Role Theory and Illness

Role Theory and Illness

A Sociological Perspective

by

Gerald Gordon, Ph.D.

University of Chicago

COLLEGE & UNIVERSITY PRESS · *Publishers*

NEW HAVEN, CONN.

TO MY MENTOR AND FRIEND

SOL LEVINE

Foreword

One of the few concepts central to medical sociology is the sick role, as central as is the concept of deviant behavior to the sociology of juvenile delinquency. This empirical study by Gordon has explored the concept of the sick role as thoroughly as ever before. Like all empirical work that is soundly based on theory, Gordon has brought Parsons' concept of the sick role to a higher level of refinement. Not only is the study of value to role theory, but it should also be of value to an understanding of how the public uses health services.

Different segments of the population vary considerably in how they regard the sick role and in turn how it initiates seeking medical care. In the physician-patient relationship this study should be of value to physicians because the general public perceives two sick roles, one in which the illness or disability has stabilized, the other in which it progresses and results in death or recovery.

The behavior of the public differs considerably in regard to these two roles, and such behavior has implications for early diagnosis and long-term rehabilitation. So, for both sociological theory and practical application, this study makes a contribution.

ODIN W. ANDERSON, PH.D.

Research Director and Professor
Center for Health Administration Studies
The University of Chicago

Acknowledgments

The author is grateful to the Health Information Foundation for its financial support of this project. Special thanks are due to Dr. John Mann and to Dr. Odin W. Anderson for their advice and moral support.

This study was also supported by National Institutes of Health Grants H-3838, M-2562, and A-2965.

Contents

I. ROLE THEORY   21

II. THE SICK ROLE   35

III. THE RESEARCH DESIGN   45

IV. CRITERIA WHICH VALIDATE THE OCCUPANCY OF THE STATUS "SICK"   49

V. BEHAVIORAL EXPECTATIONS RELEVANT TO ILLNESS   71

VI. CONCLUSIONS   97

Appendix I

Research Procedures and Methods of Analysis   105

    A. Sampling Procedure   105

    B. Plan of Analysis and Statistical Procedures   106

    C. Excerpts from Interview Manual   113

    D. Order and Method of Presentation of Questionnaire Items   116

Appendix II

Source Tables for Chapter IV   125

Appendix III

Source Tables for Chapter V   135

BIBLIOGRAPHY   151

INDEX   155

List of Tables

TABLE		PAGE
1.	Phi Coefficients for Sick–Not-Sick Matrix	52
2.	Per Cent of Persons (N=808) Who Define a Given Description as Sick or Not Sick	54
3.	Rank Order of Descriptions in Terms of Per Cent of Persons in the Low, Middle, or High Income Group Defining a Description as Sick	58
4.	Per Cent of Persons in Each Income Group Who Define a Given Description in Category 1 (Serious Prognosis) as Sick	59
5.	Per Cent of Persons in Each Income Group Who Define a Given Description in Category 2 (Favorable Prognosis) as Sick	59
6.	Per Cent of Persons in Each Income Group Who Define a Given Description in Category 3 (Functional Incapacity) as Sick	60
7.	Mean Per Cent of Sick Responses in Each Income Group to Each Anticipated Consequences Category	61
8.	Per Cent of Sick Responses in Each Income Group to Description I and Description L	61
9.	Per Cent of Sick Responses in Each Income Group to Description F and Description H	62
10.	Per Cent of Sick Responses in Each Income and Education Group to a Given Description	64
11.	Per Cent of Sick Responses in Grade School and Low-Income Groups to Descriptions D, B, and K	65

12. Per Cent of Sick Responses in College and High-Income Groups to Descriptions C and L   65

13. Per Cent of Sick Responses in Low-Income, Grade School, and Low-Income–Grade School Groups to Descriptions D, B, and K   66

14. Per Cent of Sick Responses in High-Income, College, and High-Income–College Groups to Descriptions C, L, and G   67

15. Per Cent of Persons in Low-Income–Grade School Group (N=122) Who Defined Descriptions H, F, C, and D as Sick or Not Sick   68

16. Per Cent of Sick Responses in High-Income, College, and High-Income–College Groups to Descriptions H and F   68

17. Per Cent of Persons in the Low Status and High Status Groups Who Defined Given Descriptions in Category 3 (Functional Incapacity) as Sick   69

18. Mean Per Cent of Sick Responses in the Low Status and High Status Groups to Each Anticipated Consequences Category   70

19. Tendency to Treat Ill Person as Dependent   74

20. Tendency to Treat Ill Person as Dependent When He Has Condition a, c, or d 75

21. Correlation Coefficients for Responses to Illness Conditions   77

22. Central Tendency of Responses to Conditions in Cluster 5 (Sick) and Cluster 6 (Impaired) for Each of the Four Types of Behavior   78

23. Analysis of Variance of Responses (N=808) to Illness Conditions   80

24. Mean Response by Low, Middle, and High Income Groups for Each Condition   81

25. Significance of Difference in Mean Responses of Low, Middle, and High Income Groups for Each Illness Condition   82

26. Mean Response of Low, Middle and High Income Groups to Each Illness Condition in Each Behavioral Area   84

27. Mean Response of Low, Middle and High Income Groups to Each Illness Condition in Each Behavioral Area   86

28. Mean Responses to the Behavioral Areas in Cluster 5 for Low and High Income, Education and Income–Education Groups   87

29. Mean Responses to the Behavioral Areas in Cluster 5 for Low and High Income, Education, and Income–Education Groups   88

30. Instances of Greatest Difference in Responses between Analagous Social and Economic Groups   89

31. Mean Response by Socioeconomic Status Groups for Each Condition   90

32. Mean Response to Each Dyadic Role Relationship (N=808)   94

33. Correlation Coefficients for Dyadic Role Relationships   95

34. Mean Response for Each Income Group to Each Dyadic Role Relationship   95

Introduction

Since its publication in 1950, Parsons' formulation of the sick role* has been increasingly employed by medical sociologists and others studying the sociopsychological aspects of disease. Unquestionably it has become one of the more central concepts in medical sociology. Although widely accepted, the concept is not based upon systematic observation; it has not been empirically validated nor have its key assumptions been tested. In effect, it has been accepted because of its prima facie reasonableness. In sum, we have been employing as a central concept in medical sociology a formulation developed fifteen years ago and have not, in the ensuing time, attempted to validate the concept empirically nor to develop it beyond its initial formulation. It is my belief that such an effort is long overdue and it is my hope that this work is a step in that direction.

* Talcott Parsons, *The Social System* (Glencoe, Ill.: Free Press, 1951), p. 440.

Role Theory and Illness

Chapter One

Role Theory

In studying the "sick role," we inevitably make certain assumptions about the concept of role. Since there has been considerable controversy over the analytic usefulness of the concept as well as its denotative meaning, it is important to discuss in some detail general role theory and to state explicitly how it will be used here.

The concept of role is highly useful because it offers a means of studying both the individual and the collectivity within a single conceptual framework. Social scientists, therefore, have used role theory increasingly as a major, if not central, concept in their theoretical formulations. Despite, or because of, its wide use and the numerous attempts to elaborate the various aspects of role theory, vagueness and terminological difficulties have limited its research applicability. "The concept of role remains one of the most overworked and underdeveloped in the social sciences."[1]

A major difficulty in working with the role concept arises from its interdisciplinary nature. Anthropologists, psychologists, and sociologists tend to define and clarify those aspects of role theory that are pertinent to the problems inherent in their respective disciplines. It is not that they always adhere to one analytical framework. Quite the contrary. In the first place, the

[1] Daniel J. Levinson, "Role, Personality, and Social Structure in the Organizational Setting," *Journal of Abnormal and Social Psychology,* LVIII (March, 1959), 170.

boundaries between the social sciences are vague. In addition, a great many investigators study problems of an interdisciplinary nature. Seemingly contradictory statements on role within a single work often represent shifts in research interest or analytical perspective. For example, when discussing the relationship of the individual to the social system, Parsons defines roles in terms of "reciprocal orientations."[2] Yet later in the same book, when Parsons shifts his level of analysis to the social system itself, he defines role in terms of common value orientations or standards.[3]

The interdisciplinary nature of much current social research, however, does not obviate the fact that certain aspects of role theory are more pertinent to, and have received their major emphasis in, a given social science discipline. Indeed, one might argue that there is an anthropological, a psychological, and a sociological concept of role.

In general, anthropologists have traditionally treated role as a culturally derived blueprint for behavior. In this sense it is an external constraint upon an individual and is a normative rather than a behavioral concept. Linton, in what has probably become one of the most quoted definitions of role, states:

A status, in the abstract, is a position in a particular pattern. . . . A status, as distinct from the individual who may occupy it, is simply a collection of rights and duties. Since these rights and duties can find expression only through the medium of individuals, it is extremely hard for us to maintain a distinction in our thinking between statuses and the people who hold them and exercise the rights and duties which constitute them. . . . A role represents the dynamic aspect of a status. The individual is socially assigned to a status and occupies it with relation to other statuses. When he puts the rights and duties which constitute the status into effect, he is performing a role. Role and status are quite inseparable, and the distinction between them is of only academic interest. There are no roles without statuses or statuses without roles. . . . Although all statuses and

[2] Talcott Parsons, *The Social System* (Glencoe, Ill.: Free Press, 1951), p. 26.
[3] *Ibid.*, p. 38.

roles derive from social patterns and are integral parts of patterns, they have an independent function with relation to the individuals who occupy particular statuses and exercise their role. To such individuals the combined status and role represent the minimum of attitudes and behavior which he must assume if he is to participate in the overt expression of the pattern. Status and role serve to reduce the ideal patterns for social life to individual terms. They become models for organizing the attitudes and behavior of the individual so that these will be congruous with those of the other individuals participating in the expression of the pattern.[4]

From this definition it is obvious that, while Linton recognizes a distinction between the positional referent "status" and its dynamic aspect "role," the distinction, in his own words, is of "only academic interest." Throughout his work Linton tends to use "status–role" as a unitary concept—one term invokes the other. He also fails to distinguish between the behavioral and the normative aspects of role. For instance, in his definition role apparently refers to (1) the behaviors necessary to maintain status, (2) the ideal behavior associated with a status, and (3) the actual behavior that results from occupying a status.

The failure to differentiate clearly the various elements of role theory is a result of the anthropologist's assumptions and problems. A prime concern of anthropologists has been the description of societies on a macrocultural level. Murdock states that, in addition to reporting on a specific area of interest, the anthropologist is expected to prepare "a descriptive account as complete as he can make it of the entire culture of the people studied."[5] Since it is important to describe a culture as it actually exists, anthropologists must abstract a cultural construct which, while it may "not be in exact correspondence with the real cul-

[4] Ralph Linton, *The Study of Man* (New York: D. Appleton-Century Co., 1936), pp. 113-14.

[5] George P. Murdock, "Sociology and Anthropology," in John Gillin (ed.), *For a Science of Social Man* (New York: Macmillan Co., 1954), p. 21, as quoted in N. Gross, W. S. Mason and A. W. McEachern, *Explorations in Role Analysis* (New York: John Wiley & Sons, Inc., 1958), p. 22.

ture at any point . . . provides a brief and convenient approxima-
tion of the conditions existing within the real culture."[6]

In macrocultural descriptions of small societies the distinctions
between role and status, between behavior and expectation, may
well have been "academic." Indeed, a more complicated classifi-
cation system might have hindered rather than aided the anthropologist. This formulation, however, has several limitations
when applied to the analysis of other types of social phenomena.
There is an implicit assumption that there exists a uniform mode
of behavior in regard to status. Descriptions based on such
constructs tend to minimize or not to treat systematic variations
in status–role behavior. But understanding the factors that cause
these variations is particularly important in complex societies
such as the United States where, as Gross, Mason, and Mc-
Eachern point out, consensus concerning status–role behavior is
often lacking and where multimodal patterns of behavior in
regard to a status occur.[7] Despite these and other criticisms,
Linton's conception of role is probably the most widely known
and influential in the social sciences.[8]

The psychologist, on the other hand, is primarily interested in
increasing his understanding of individual behavior. Cultural and
social phenomena are peripheral interests and are relevant only
insofar as they relate to individual behavior. As a consequence
he generally employs role as a mediating factor between social
system pressures and individual behavior. This has led to a
different approach to role theory. For instance, compare Sarbin's
treatment of role with that of Linton:

> In role theory, the person as the broad sociological unit
> of interaction is retained, but a somewhat finer unit, the

[6] Ralph Linton, *The Cultural Background of Personality* (New York:
D. Appleton-Century Co., 1945), pp. 42-43.

[7] Gross, Mason, and McEachern, *op. cit.*, p. 25.

[8] On the basis of their summary of role literature, Neiman and Hughes
concluded that "there is an increasing trend toward associating the concept
role with that of status. Here [Linton's] perhaps is one of the most
definitive uses of the concept—the one about which there is the most
consensus." Lionel J. Neiman and James W. Hughes, "The Problem of the
Concept of Role—A Survey of the Literature," *Social Forces*, XXX
(December, 1951), 149.

role, is added. Thus role theory embraces reciprocal action between persons, but these actions are organized into roles. If this were the only addition, we would have no more than an extension of traditional sociological theory. A second kind of interaction has been added, however, which marks role theory as a unique social psychological formulation, namely, the interaction of role and self. Such a theory aims at problems (at the third of Murphy's levels of complexity), where there is structure within the organism and structure within the environment. It is to the investigation of these structures and their interaction that role theory addresses itself. In broad perspective, contemporary role theory regards human conduct as the product of the interaction of self and role. (Not dissimilar is Parsons and Shils' idea of need dispositions and role expectations (1951)).[9]

Sarbin's position, relating the concepts of self and role (the interactional position), has a long tradition in psychology. It is found in embryonic form as early as 1892 in William James's *Psychology.* But it remained for George Herbert Mead to develop a detailed system of the interrelationship between self and role. Mead defined "self" as the capacity of mind and organism "to be an object to itself."[10] The self is the result of the organism's ability to evaluate itself as a social object. Such evaluation occurs when an individual responds to his own gestures in terms of the response which he feels his gesture would elicit in another.

Within Mead's interactional framework, even strictly individualistic, biological reactions, such as elimination, posture, locomotion, and sleep, become socialized or conditioned through the tuition of others. The maturing child builds into his own stimulus –response system the responses of others (directed toward him). The child can then call out another's responses toward him and can in turn take the role of a specific other. Mead explains this process as follows:

[9] Theodore R. Sarbin, "Role Theory," in Gardner Lindzey (ed.), *Handbook of Social Psychology* (Cambridge, Mass.: Addison-Wesley Publishing Co., 1954), p. 223.

[10] George Herbert Mead, *Mind, Self, and Society* (Chicago: University of Chicago Press, 1952), p. 136.

The illustration used was of a person playing baseball. Each one of his own acts is determined by his assumption of the action of the others who are playing the game. What he does is controlled by his being everyone else on that team, at least insofar as those attitudes affect his own particular response.[11]

Mead has had great influence in many areas of psychology. Psychologists such as Cameron, Sargent, McClelland, Sarbin, Sullivan, and others lean heavily upon his interactional theory.

Another group of psychologists, while maintaining an interest in the self concept, has focused upon the interrelationship of role and the generically more inclusive concept of personality. Newcomb, a leading proponent of this position, states:

> From the point of view of personality the individual's relation to society is best described in terms of his attitudes toward other people who have certain role expectations towards him. From the point of view of culture, his relation to society is described in terms of the degree to which and the ways in which he deviates from the prescribed roles. From either point of view, personality and prescribed roles are interdependent.[12]

Whether he is interested in role in relation to the self or in relation to the more inclusive personality system, the psychologist's unit of analysis is the individual and his objective is an explanation of individual behavior. Role and status are, therefore, external and auxiliary rather than central concepts. They are not, however, unimportant concepts; the quantity of work by psychologists that has dealt with role and status gives ample evidence of the importance they attach to these concepts. But the psychologist qua psychologist has tended to treat role and status as a given and not as a variable for study. In this context it is interesting to note that in *Mind, Self, and Society,* there is no index reference to either status or position. Aside from stating that role is social in nature and analogous to the rules of a

---

[11] *Ibid.,* p. 154.

[12] Theodore M. Newcomb, *Social Psychology* (New York: Dryden Press, 1951), p. 414.

game, Mead does not discuss or define role as such. Moreover, in the quotation from Sarbin, there is no mention of status or of the determinants of role content.

The failure to emphasize these concepts is neither an oversight nor a lack of knowledge; it indicates instead that these aspects of the status–role concept are not central to the psychologist's interests. Having little interest in the status–role concept as such, he treats positional referents, role content, status interrelationships, and the like, as non-problematic. On the other hand, the psychologist has devoted a great deal of attention to delineating and developing such concepts as role-taking, role-playing, role conflict, generalized other, etc., which, being clearly relevant to individual behavioral variations, are central to his level of analysis and interests. Given the historical development of role theory within psychology and the psychologist's areas of concern, this treatment of role has been not only extremely useful but more or less inevitable.

It is more difficult to delineate the sociologist's areas of interest. Conflicting opinion on the nature and data of sociology are rife in the writings of its founders. Comte viewed sociology primarily as a tool for the perfection of society; Spencer felt that, while the sociologist should study social evolution, he could not and should not interfere with the evolutionary process.[13] Weber and Durkheim differed sharply on the sociologist's level of analysis. Weber believed that *verstehen,* or understanding, on a personal or psychological level was essential to social analysis,[14] while Durkheim vigorously argued that sociology should deal only with "social facts," which he described as constraints upon behavior that are external to the individual and hence not reducible to individual consciousness.[15]

In one form or another, this conflict in viewpoint affects the works of many contemporary sociologists. Parsons, for instance, has sought to develop a conceptual framework for understanding

[13] Harry Elmer Barnes, *An Introduction to the History of Sociology* (Chicago: University of Chicago Press, 1948), p. 81.

[14] Talcott Parsons, "Max Weber's Sociological Analysis of Capitalism and Modern Institutions," in Barnes, *op. cit.,* p. 291.

[15] Emile Durkheim, *Suicide* (Glencoe, Ill.: Free Press, 1951), pp. 35-39.

social phenomena without regard to specific social contents or problems; but Mills insists that sociology should concern itself with meaningful social problems. Mills also criticizes the work of sociologists such as Lazarsfeld who have conducted attitude studies from what in Mills's opinion is a psychologistic viewpoint. Mills points out that, as a historical doctrine, psychologism

> rests upon an explicit metaphysical denial of the reality of social structures. In a still more general way, and of more direct interest to our concern with the current research policies of social science, psychologism rests upon the idea that if we study a series of individuals and their milieux, the results of our studies in some way can be added up to knowledge of social structure.[16]

Explicit in the writings of these and other sociologists, however, is the belief that the sociologist should study phenomena which are social in nature and occur within the framework of a social system. This belief has meant, in effect, that sociologists, whatever their philosophical or methodological orientation, have for the most part concentrated upon a subject area which is larger than the individual but less than, or asymptotic to, the entire social system. Recently, some agreement has emerged among many sociologists that the unit of analysis that is most meaningfully related to this general area is the "reciprocal relationship," the socially preconditioned interaction of two or more persons. Loomis, for example, calls the reciprocal relationship the "core datum of sociology."[17]

[16] C. Wright Mills, *The Sociological Imagination* (New York: Oxford University Press, 1959), p. 67.

[17] The following describes reciprocal relationship more fully: "The more specialized frame of reference of sociology is limited to reciprocal action or interaction. Interaction as a special type of action (or activity, terms which are here used as synonymous) loses none of the aforementioned attributes of activity, but is distinguished by additional attributes. The separate activities of the actors involved in a particular case of interaction are not sufficient to explain the 'meaning' of the interaction. The meaning lies not in the unit acts of the participating actors but in the interaction itself which constitutes a legitimate and important subject of study, and in its own right becomes the specialized phenomena with which sociology deals. 'Interaction,' the core datum of sociology, has been defined as 'any event by which one party tangibly influences the overt actions or the state of

Paralleling the emphasis on reciprocity as the core datum of sociological analysis has been the emergence of functionalism as a major methodological approach. In essence, the reciprocal–functional orientation focuses upon factors related to the functions, changes, and maintenance of the reciprocal relationship, both in terms of its own dynamics and in terms of the larger systems of which it is a part. Parsons, who has identified himself with the reciprocal–functional position, states:

> Sociology is clearly concerned with the observation and analysis of human social behavior, that is, the interaction of pluralities of human beings, the forms their relationships take, and a variety of the conditions and determinants of these forms and of changes in them.[18]

The impact of functionalism upon all aspects of sociological investigation has been so widespread that Davis questions whether one is still justified in referring to functionalism as a unique methodological position, for with the growth of methodological sophistication, one can no longer distinguish functionalism from sociological analysis per se. He states:

> One should first realize that consensus on the definition of structural–functional analysis does not exist, but that examination of the features most commonly mentioned and of the work actually done under the label shows it to be, in effect, synonymous with sociological analysis.[19]

Not all sociologists agree, however, that reciprocal relationships are the core data of sociology, nor do they all hold the functionalist position. Mills and Sorokin, for instance, adhere to an institutional–historical frame of reference. Furthermore,

mind of the other.' It is a reciprocal and interdependent activity, designated as having the equality of complementarity or double contingency." Charles P. Loomis, *Social Systems* (Princeton: D. Van Nostrand Co., 1960), p. 3.

[18] Talcott Parsons, "Psychology and Sociology," in Gillin, *op. cit.*, p. 68.

[19] Kingsley Davis, "The Myth of Functional Analysis as a Special Method in Sociology and Anthropology," *American Sociological Review*, XXIV (December, 1959), 757.

even the advocates of the reciprocal–functional position differ in their interests and their approach to problems. Nevertheless, the great number of articles and books written from a reciprocal–functional position indicate that it has provided a valuable orientation for a great many sociologists.

In short, while other sociological orientations have their advocates, the reciprocal–functional orientation appears to have the most acceptance among sociologists. This dual orientation almost axiomatically draws one's attention to the how and why of the reciprocal relationship in the larger social system.

 Within the reciprocal relationship, the key factors of the functions, maintenance, and changes are the social identities (status and role) of the participants. Status and role provide the means by which individuals are able to engage in reciprocal activity. They are at one and the same time the cues for and the predeterminers of behavior. Status and role are in effect the building blocks of the reciprocal relationship.

Questions about status and role from this perspective must of necessity differ from those asked by the anthropologist and psychologist. Bates, for example, points to the following as major sociological concerns that cannot be adequately treated within the framework of anthropological or psychological conceptions of role:

1. The concept of social position or social status (only position will be used hereafter) as usually defined does not allow adequate description and analysis of the internal structure of a position. At present it is possible only to state that a position is a location in a social structure which is associated with a set of norms called rights and duties and to which is attached a certain amount of prestige—no systematic means of describing the relationship between the norms and other elements which compose a situation.

2. The present concepts of position and role do not allow the analyst to deal with problems of real behavior in an adequate fashion. About all that he can do using these concepts is to state that the norms which are associated with a position influence the behavior of a person occupying the position. How they influence particular parts of that be-

havior has been more or less neglected especially in present theory.

3. The present concept makes it very difficult to conduct an analysis which deals with more than two positions. Since positions are conceived of as coming in reciprocally related pairs, the concept has proved difficult to apply to anything larger than a dyad—as a consequence little actual research in the area of group structure has been done using the ideas of social position as a primary tool of analysis.[20]

In the past, whether because of the historical development of role or the lack of agreement about the sociologist's areas of concern, a conception of role relevant to his problems has been lacking in his work. Of course, sociologists have employed role and allied concepts widely, but they have tended to employ them in either their anthropological or their psychological contexts. In a recently published sociological textbook, for example, role is defined in an anthropological context.

> Each of these statuses carries with it a set of rules or norms which prescribe how the person who occupies it should or should not behave under particular circumstances. That cluster of norms we call a "role." Status and role are thus two sides of a single coin. Status is a socially identified position; role is the pattern of behavior expected of persons who occupy a particular status.[21]

In another widely used textbook role is defined in a psychological context:

> How an individual actually performs in a given position as distinct from how he is supposed to perform, we call his role. The role then is the manner in which a person actually carries out the requirement of his position. It is the dynamic aspect of status or office and as such is always influenced by factors other than the stipulations of the position itself.[22]

[20] Frederick L. Bates, "Position, Role, and Status: A Reformulation of Concepts," *Social Forces*, XXXIV (May, 1956), 313.

[21] Ely Chinoy, *Society* (New York: Random House, 1961), p. 29.

[22] Kingsley Davis, *Human Society* (New York: Macmillan Co., 1949), p. 90.

These conceptions not only lack relevance for the sociologist, they have severely limited the areas of sociological investigation. Specifically, anthropological and psychological conceptions of role make it difficult to deal with the structural necessities of ongoing social systems and their functional consequences.

Recognizing that anthropological and psychological conceptions of role have, at best, limited usefulness in a sociological context, many sociologists have sought to develop role conceptions more pertinent to their interests. Notable work in this direction has been done by Levinson; Goode; Turner; Gross, Mason, and McEachern; Bates; and others. Sociological role conceptions are concerned largely with clear and precise differentiations between status and role. Furthermore, these reformulations are characterized by the assumptions that status and role are not "two sides of a single coin" and that variations in the nature and complexity of the reciprocal relationship are related to variations in status–role expectations. Bates, for instance, working with these three basic concepts:

1. *Position:* A location in a social structure which is associated with a set of social norms;

2. *Role:* A part of a social position consisting of a more–less integrated or related sub-set of social norms which is distinguishable from other sets of norms forming the same position;

3. *Norm:* A patterned or commonly held behavior expectation—a learned response, held in common by members of a social group;[23]

develops the following postulates concerning role and status (position):

Post. 1. Within any given culture there exists a limited number of roles which were combined in various ways to compose a limited number of positions.

Post. 2. Within any given position there tends to be a strain towards consistency or adjustment between the various roles composing a position.

---

[23] Bates, *op. cit.,* p. 314.

Post. 3. Each position contains certain dominant roles to which are adjusted certain recessive roles.

Post. 4. No role exists without a paired reciprocal role which is a part of a different position.[24]

Gross, Mason, and McEachern, whose work appears to have developed logically from Bates, have refined Bates's original conceptions of position, role, and norm. In addition, they have treated role sanctions in detail and have clearly set out the differences between role expectation and role behavior.

In examining several role conceptions, I have become convinced that no single one is relevant to all types of behavioral phenomena. Indeed, the usefulness of any of these three conceptions is restricted to the specific problems and levels of analysis. When these conceptions are used, it is important to recognize their limitations. Unfortunately, many investigators have considered one or the other definitive and the ensuing verbiage has hindered the development of a truly interdisciplinary status–role theory.

Since my primary interest in studying the sick role is sociological, the conceptions of status and role used in this paper naturally follow closely those developed by Gross, Mason, and McEachern. But aside from my personal interests, if the sick role as an analytic concept is to become more useful, that role must be studied in terms of the constraints and problems imposed by sociological analysis. In short, because I am interested in certain questions and because I feel that there have been specific gaps in the development of the sick role concept, the discriminations and definitions I have employed throughout this study are sociological rather than psychological or anthropological.

[24] *Ibid.*, pp. 315-17.

Chapter Two

The Sick Role

It has long been recognized that the sick person occupies a unique social position: he is freed from daily activities, and he is dependent upon others for his well-being. Only with the publication of Parsons' *The Social System*,[1] however, has the concept of the sick role gained prominence and become widely recognized as a viable tool in social analysis. Parsons' contributions were essentially the crystallization of latent conceptions of the sick person and the setting forth of an ideal system by which behavior could be judged. In this connection, Freidson states:

> A rather popular way of conceptualizing the doctor–patient relationship lies in constructing a formal model based on how physician and patient *should* behave. This sort of model underlies much of the hortatory writing of professionals about themselves and their patients. In a more neutral, elegant, and empirically useful way it also forms the basis for Talcott Parsons' analysis. . . . The virtue of this kind of analysis is that it provides us with a definition of (philosophically) the "essence" of the relationship. We may use it as a fixed standard by which we may measure the variable deviations of reality. However, it cannot really explain reality. It can only say what reality should be and note exceptions: it can note that the patient should submit to professional authority but, in fact, does not.[2]

Conservative

[1] Talcott Parsons, *The Social System* (Glencoe, Ill.: Free Press, 1951).

[2] Eliot Freidson, *Patients' Views of Medical Practice* (New York: Russell Sage Foundation, 1961), p. 190.

liberal

35

Because of the broad influence of Parsons' formulation of the sick role, a meaningful exploration of role theory and illness behavior must begin with an understanding of his conceptual framework. In order to provide a referent for further discussion, let us briefly summarize Parsons' sick role concept.

Parsons deals primarily with three areas: role relationships, behavioral presumptions, and reactions to illness.

A. *Role relationships.*—The major dyadic role relationship in Parsons' framework is that between the physician and the patient. Parsons states:

> The immediately relevant social structures consist in the patterning of the role of the medical practitioner himself and though to common sense it may seem superfluous to analyze it that of the sick person himself.[3]

Modifying and acting upon this relationship is the family, and Parsons goes on to say:

> The need of help is also just as strong because the solidarity of the family imposes a very strong pressure on the healthy members to see that the sick one gets the best possible care. It is, indeed, very common if not usual for the pressure of family members to tip the balance in the admission of being sick enough to go to bed or call a doctor, when the patient himself could tend to stay out longer.[4]

B. *Behavioral presumptions.*—Parsons posits four aspects of the sick role:

1. The sick person is exempt from social responsibility.

First, is the exemption from normal social role responsibilities, which of course is relative to the nature and severity of the illness. This exemption requires legitimation by and to the various alters involved and the physician often serves as a court of appeal as well as a direct legitimatizing agent. It is noteworthy that like all institutionalized patterns the legitimation of being sick enough to avoid obligations

---

[3] Parsons, *op. cit.*, pp. 433-34.
[4] *Ibid.*, p. 446.

can not only be a right of the sick person but an obligation upon him. People are often resistant to admitting they are sick and it is not uncommon for others to tell them that they *ought* to stay in bed. The word generally has a moral connotation. It goes almost without saying that this legitimation has the social function of protection against "malingering."[5]

2. The sick person cannot be expected to take care of himself.

The second closely related aspect is the institutionalized definition that the sick person cannot be expected by "pulling himself together" to get well by an act of decision or will. In this sense also he is exempted from responsibility—he is in a condition that must "be taken care of." Of course the process of recovery may be spontaneous but while the illness lasts he can't "help it." This element in the definition of the state of illness is obviously crucial as a bridge to the acceptance of "help."[6]

3. The sick person should want to get well.

The third element is the definition of the state of being ill as itself undesirable with its obligation to want to "get well." The first two elements of legitimation of the sick role thus are conditional in a highly important sense. It is a relative legitimation so long as he is in this unfortunate state which both he and alter hope he can get out of as expeditiously as possible.[7]

4. The sick person should seek medical advice and cooperate with medical experts.

Finally, the fourth closely related element is the obligation —in proportion to the severity of the condition, of course—to seek *technically competent* help, namely, in the most usual case, that of a physician and to *cooperate* with him in the process of trying to get well. It is here, of course, that the role of the sick person as the patient becomes articulated with that of the physician in a complementary role structure.[8]

[5] *Ibid.*, pp. 436-37.
[6] *Ibid.*, p. 437.
[7] *Ibid.*
[8] *Ibid.*

C. *Other reactions to illness.*—Parsons states, however, that because of the severe anxiety and strain produced by an illness the sick role may be rejected and other reactions occur. He feels that often the sick person will deny that he is ill or will give in to a feeling of total helplessness and demand excessive care and attention:

> Perhaps the most definite point is that for the "normal" person illness, the more so the greater its severity, constitutes a frustration of expectancies of his normal life pattern. He is cut off from his normal spheres of activity, and many of his normal enjoyments. He is often humiliated by his incapacity to function normally. His social relationships are disrupted to a greater or a less degree. He may have to bear discomfort or pain which is hard to bear, and he may have to face serious alterations of his prospects for the future, in the extreme but by no means uncommon case the termination of his life. . . . Therefore even the necessary degree of emotional acceptance of the reality is difficult. One very possible reaction is to attempt to deny illness or various aspects of it, to refuse to "give in" to it. Another may be exaggerated self-pity and whining, a complaining demand for more help than is necessary or feasible, especially for incessant personal attention.[9]

Although Parsons recognizes that people differ in their reactions to illness, he attributes such differences to variations in emotional response. Whenever responses differ from those that Parsons has postulated, they are viewed as deviations from a norm. When Freidson states, "We may use it [Parsons' formulation] as a fixed standard by which we may measure the variable deviation from reality,"[10] he draws attention to the unimodal nature of the formulation. One consequence of the assumption of unimodality is that variations in role conception will likely be attributed to psychological rather than to social factors, and the possibility that such variations are structurally related to the social system is either neglected or denied.

Unimodal conceptions of role, while hindering social investiga-

[9] *Ibid.*, p. 443.
[10] Freidson, *op. cit.*, p. 190.

tions are, as I have shown in the preceding chapter, useful in anthropological and psychological research. For instance, the psychologist can, indeed must, treat the context of the sick role as non-problematic. Parsons' development of the sick role is therefore extremely useful to him. As Gross, Mason, and McEachern point out, conceptualizations of status and role based upon Linton's assumption of unimodality relate

> . . . the basic ideas of social structure and culture in a form in which they could be readily assimilated into existing social–psychological conceptual schemes. It brought culture and social structure down to the individual level, to the level of analysis at which the psychologist feels most comfortable in developing theory and treating data. The relevance of the broad, and to many psychologists the vague, ideas of culture and social organization to their problems became more evident.[11]

It is not surprising therefore to discover that sociologists have used Parsons' formulation in studies that are primarily anthropological or psychological. For example, Rose Coser,[12] employs the sick role as an anthropological concept, while Mechanic and Volkart[13] employ it as a psychological concept. Nor is it surprising to note that relatively little of the reported research falls within the context which I have defined as sociological. For instance, neither in the *Sociological Abstracts* (1957-61) nor in recent surveys of research (*Sociological Studies of Health and Sickness;*[14] *Sociology Today;*[15] *Patients, Physicians and Illness*[16])

[11] N. Gross, W. S. Mason, A. W. McEachern, *Explorations in Role Analysis* (New York: John Wiley & Sons Inc., 1958), p. 331.

[12] Rose Coser, "A Home Away from Home," in Dorrian Apple (ed.), *Sociological Studies of Health and Sickness* (New York: McGraw-Hill Book Co., 1960).

[13] David Mechanic and Edmund A. Volkart, "Stress, Illness Behavior, and the Sick Role," *American Sociological Review,* XXVI (February, 1961), 51-58.

[14] Apple, *op. cit.*

[15] Robert K. Merton, Leonard Broom, and Leonard S. Cottrell, Jr. (eds.), *Sociology Today* (New York: Basic Books, 1959).

[16] E. Gartly Jaco (ed.), *Patients, Physicians and Illness* (Glencoe, Ill.: Free Press, 1958).

arc there any references to studies treating the sick role as a sociological variable. As Irving K. Zola, in a recent review of the literature states:

> It has been left for the most part to anthropologists and workers in the field of mental health to discuss the differing conceptions of, responses to, and concern with medically serious symptoms and relate these not only to each other but also to the seeking of medical aid.[17]

The use of the sick role in anthropological and psychological studies and its limited use in sociological research is due partly to a temporal constraint implicit in role analysis, namely, that before one can examine "reality," one must have a relatively simple standard by which to judge behavior. The initial development of a role is therefore usually based on a highly abstracted cultural or social system and predicated on the assumption that roles are unimodal. This development serves both as the base for future anthropological and psychological investigations and as a necessary prerequisite for sociological research. For through the existence of a fixed standard researchers become attuned to patterned variations in role conception; these systematic variations in role draw attention to the fact that an individual's role and role behavior are not only related to his position in a given relationship, but are also related to his position vis-à-vis the ongoing social system. For instance, Freidson comments on the limitations of Parsons' formulations:

> In order to understand and predict the chances that an expectation will be met, then, it is not enough to specify the expectations of everyone included in the doctor's or patients' role-set. Attention must be paid to the social structure in which those perspectives are located, and there must be systematic specification of the variable situations and positions of influences in which doctors and patients find themselves.[18]

---

[17] Irving K. Zola, "Socio-cultural Factors in the Seeking of Medical Aid" (Massachusetts General Hospital, mimeographed), p. 5.

[18] Freidson, *op. cit.*, p. 191.

Of course these stages are not mutually exclusive. Quite the contrary. I am, however, stating that a degree of anthropological and psychological conceptualization and work is normally a necessity for treating a given role in a sociological context.

The problems that arise in the use of a unimodal concept lead to a questioning of that concept. Paradoxically, the usefulness and authoritativeness of the unimodal concept can delay the investigation of the basic assumptions underlying the concept, as is particularly the case with the sick role. The widespread acceptance of Parsons' formulation by well-known sociologists has given it an authoritative aura. It has become legitimized in a sense through repetition. For example, despite evidence presented by investigators such as Saunders,[19] Koos,[20] and Nett,[21] among others, to the effect that expectations regarding illness vary from group to group, Loomis in a recent sociological text presents Parsons' formulation of the sick role with only minor qualifications.[22] And only in the last few years have investigators (e.g., Gilliam, DeGroot, and Marx;[23] Kasselbaum;[24] and Baumann[25]) begun to view the sick role from what I have defined as a sociological perspective.

Parsons' conception of the sick role has, of course, been useful to medical sociologists, but its untested assumptions and lack of empirical validation limit its future usefulness. Con-

[19] Lyle Saunders, *Cultural Difference and Medical Care* (New York: Russell Sage Foundation, 1954), pp. 5-6.

[20] Earl Lomon Koos, "Illness in Regionville," in Apple, *op. cit.*, pp. 9-14.

[21] Emily M. Nett, "Some Social and Psychological Correlates of Attitudes toward Medical Doctors" (paper presented at the annual meeting of the American Sociological Society, Washington, D.C., August, 1957), pp. 1-8.

[22] Charles P. Loomis, *Social Systems* (Princeton: D. Van Nostrand Co., 1960), p. 311.

[23] Sylvia B. Gilliam, Ida DeGroot, and John H. Marx, "Operationalization of the Theoretical Framework for the Study of Patterns of Medical Care" (Working Paper II, mimeographed), pp. 15-18.

[24] Gene G. Kasselbaum and Barbara Baumann, "Dimensions of the Sick Role" (Cornell University Medical College, mimeographed).

[25] Barbara Baumann, "Diversities in Conceptions of Health and Physical Fitness," *Journal of Health and Human Behavior*, II (Spring, 1961), 39-46.

sequently, it is necessary to determine the extent to which Parsons' description of sick role expectations is valid. Equally important is whether these expectations are affected by sociocultural variations. In sum, I am asking whether one can predict a person's behavioral expectations regarding a relationship (i.e., doctor–patient) from knowing his position (status) in that relationship, or whether such prediction depends upon identifying his position vis-à-vis the social system as well.

Furthermore, if we are to predict illness behavior, we must determine not only the behavioral expectations associated with the sick role but also the conditions under which the expectations become operative. Therefore, with respect to Parsons' insights, the following variables and hypotheses[26] were investigated:

I.   Criteria that determine whether or not a person may occupy the status "sick."

    A.   Functional or physical incapacities:

        Hypothesis 1—There is an inverse relationship between socioeconomic status and the importance of functional or physical incapacity as a factor identifying someone as sick.

    B.   The role of the physician as a legitimizing agent:

        Hypothesis 2—In the absence of physical and functional incapacity, there is a direct relationship between socioeconomic status and the tendency to define someone as sick on the basis of his being under a physician's care.

    C.   Anticipated consequences:

        Hypothesis 3—The poorer or more uncertain the prognosis, the greater the tendency to define someone as sick.

II.   Behavioral expectations regarding an ill person.

    A.   Dependency patterns: In my examination of role expectations regarding an ill person, I have followed Parsons' lead in concentrating on the three aspects of

---

[26] The hypotheses listed are not part of any theoretical approach. Their use is analogous to questions for investigation.

role expectations which he feels are important in the sick role.

    1. Expectations regarding social responsibility.

    2. Expectations regarding patient care.
       a) Information.
       b) Physical comfort.

    3. Expectations regarding technically competent help.

Hypothesis 4—As prognosis varies from controlled and known to unknown and serious, the tendency increases to exempt the ill person from social responsibility and from care of self, and to insure his obtaining technically competent help (i.e., the person will be treated as a dependent).

Hypothesis 5—Except in severe cases of functional and physical impairment, prognosis will be a more important factor than incapacity in determining the response towards the ill person.

Hypothesis 6—As socioeconomic status decreases, there is a greater likelihood that persons having illness with a non-serious prognosis will be treated as dependent.

B.   Dyadic role relations: Continuing on the path set by Parsons, the three dyadic role relations that he feels are important were examined in terms of the four reactions which he postulates occur when a person is sick:

       doctor–patient,
       family–patient, and
       self (ego)–patient

    1. Reactions to illness
       a) Overindependence.—tendency to demand more independence when sick than when well.
       b) Normal independence.—tendency to seek to maintain as far as possible the responsibilities inherent in the status "well."

c) Dependence.—tendency to give up some responsibility but with a residue of responsibility remaining (Parsons' sick role).

d) Self-pity.—tendency to view one's self as helpless and to reject the possibility of self-help.

Hypothesis 7—When a person is defined as sick, a high correlation will exist between the dependency or independency pattern in one dyadic relationship and that of the other dyadic relationships.

Hypothesis 8—As socioeconomic status decreases, the tendency to regard independence as the appropriate behavior of the sick person in each of the three dyadic role relationships increases.

Chapter Three

The Research Design

Aims

The aims of this investigation were (1) to examine the validity of the sick-role concept as developed by Parsons with particular reference to his assumption of unimodality, and (2) to examine variations in behavioral expectations relating to illness within different dyadic relationships.

Questionnaire

The questionnaire used in the interviewing was completed after three pretests. It was translated into Spanish to permit adequate interviewing of Spanish-speaking respondents. The interviews averaged a little over two and a half hours.

The questionnaire covered major areas believed to be related to sick-role expectations as well as more general health areas. The specific nature and type of question was governed by previous conceptualization of the sick role and by the results of the pretests. The following is a brief outline of the areas covered that are relevant to this study.

I. Attitudes regarding illness and the sick role.

    A. A series of questions to ascertain the respondent's definition of health and causes of illness: When does he think somebody is sick? What can be done to maintain health? What is covered by the word "healthy"?

B. A series of questions to establish how the respondent feels about being sick: Does he find some aspects pleasant and others intolerable? How does he visualize his life as a sick person? What does he expect in the way of treatment from his family and from physicians? How does he think he should act?

II. Demographic data. A description of the respondent and his family: income, occupation, size of family, ethnic background, age, sex, education, information on main wage-earner, religion, languages spoken in home, etc.

Interviewing

In any large-scale interviewing, the researcher must rely on many other persons to obtain his information. Even with excellent interviewers and extensive training, it is impossible to reproduce laboratory conditions and present each respondent with identical stimuli; the personalities, styles of presentation, and physical factors of the interviewers are impossible to control. The time and the setting of the interview are controlled by the respondent rather than the researcher. In one situation, a baby may interrupt an interview; in another, a wife, despite the efforts of the interviewer, may insist on correcting her husband's responses. Thus, in large-scale interviewing, stimuli will not remain constant under the best of circumstances. Researchers basing their findings on large-scale interviewing must assume, therefore, that the variation in stimuli will be random and will not introduce a bias in the data. But unless great care is taken in the selection, training, and supervision of interviewers, this assumption is untenable. Not only do interviewers vary in competence, but the training received by interviewers varies in quality.

The interviewers used in this study were given extensive training in interviewing in general and in the specific procedures relevant to this study.[1] Each interviewer was required to complete one sample interview and then go over the questionnaire with a senior member of the research staff. This procedure was

---

[1] For additional information, see excerpts from interview manual, Appendix I, pp. 113-15.

repeated until the senior staff member felt the interviewer was ready to carry on alone. Senior staff members contacted 10 per cent of the persons interviewed to check on the accuracy and quality of the interviewing. If there were major discrepancies or the interviewing seemed poor, the interview was voided, and that interviewer's entire work was reappraised.

Sampling

The universe of inquiry consists of an area probability sample of one thousand persons residing in New York City during 1957-58. Eighty-one per cent (808 persons) of our potential sample were interviewed. No persons in the armed forces were interviewed. No persons under twenty-one years of age going to school full time, and hence dependent, were interviewed. No persons momentarily at the interviewing address but in fact residing at some other address were interviewed.[2]

The representativeness of the data is, therefore, limited to New York City (excluding Staten Island). But, as Eysenck points out,[3] even when a sample is totally non-representative, the patterns of interrelationship remain valid and can be extended to groups other than that represented by the sample.[4]

[2] For details of sampling procedure, see Appendix I, pp. 105-6.

[3] H. J. Eysenck, "Primary Social Attitudes—A Comparison of Attitude Patterns in England, Germany and Sweden," *Journal of Abnormal and Social Psychology*, XLVIII (1953), 567.

[4] For the detailed plan of analysis and statistical procedures, see Appendix I, pp. 106-13.

Chapter Four

Criteria Which Validate the Occupancy of the Status 'Sick'

Sickness as a medical phenomenon differs from sickness as a social phenomenon. Socially, a person is "sick" only when one or more others identify and treat him as sick. Sociologists have recently begun to study the criteria which serve to validate socially the status "sick." Not only has there been little research done in this area, but the value of the research findings is frequently limited by the nature of the sample (i.e., purposive or non-representative samples). For example, in her study, "How Laymen Define Illness," Apple used a sample consisting of sixty persons residing in the Boston area.[1] The sample, however, contained only "four blue-collar workers."[2] And Mechanic, in his study of validating criteria, used a sample consisting solely of college students.[3] While samples of this type do not allow the

[1] Dorrian Apple, "How Laymen Define Illness," *Journal of Health and Human Behavior*, I (Fall, 1960), 219–25.

[2] *Ibid.*, p. 221.

[3] David Mechanic, "The Concept of Illness Behavior," *Journal of Chronic Diseases*, XV (February, 1962), 189–94.

investigator to make extensive generalizations about population parameters or to undertake an extensive socioeconomic analysis, they do enable him to identify the criteria which are important in validating the status "sick." Thus, despite the analytical limitations resulting from their samples, researchers such as Apple and Mechanic provide strong evidence that the following four factors play an important role:

1. *Legitimization by physician:* Someone is under a doctor's care.

2. *Symptoms:* Pains, discomforts, or other manifestations that indicate a change in health.

3. *Functional incapacity:* The inability of persons to perform normal work activities.

4. *Prognosis:* The expected outcome of the illness, i.e., probably get worse, get better, stabilize, uncertain, etc.

In order to explore the manner and extent to which these four factors serve to validate occupancy of the status "sick," we described the health of various persons to our respondents and then asked them to state whether the persons described were "sick" or "not sick." Because of time limitations and respondents' resistance during the pretest, we were obliged to limit our descriptions to twelve out of the one hundred or so possible permutations of these four factors and the qualitative differences within each factor. The following twelve descriptions were chosen because they appeared most relevant to the hypothesis concerning validation of the sick role.

Descriptions of Illness States

A. Has a severe case of pneumonia.
   (Validating factors: Implies a medical diagnosis, symptoms, functional incapacity, and uncertain prognosis.)

B. Had something a year ago and as a result lost the use of his legs.
   (Validating factors: Person had an illness which left him with a severe handicap.)

C. Is recovering but not yet back to work.
(Validating factors: Person is recovering, but not yet able to function. The implication, however, is that he will go back to work.)

D. Had something five years ago and since then cannot do strenuous work.
(Validating factors: Some work is still possible, but person is unable to do hard work.)

E. Has persistent pains in the stomach but can still work.
(Validating factors: Symptoms exist, but function is not impaired, uncertainty about cause.)

F. Has had arthritis for the past several years.
(Validating factors: Medical definition is given, symptoms exist, no indication of future prognosis.)

G. Is under a doctor's care but can work.
(Validating factors: Person is under care of a physician, but no symptoms are mentioned and there is no functional impairment.)

H. Has increasingly bad attacks of rheumatism.
(Validating factors: Repeat of F with the added factor of worsening prognosis.)

I. Has an illness which keeps him in bed on and off. It has gotten worse, there appears little hope that it will improve.
(Validating factors: Illness which prevents person from functioning, worsening or uncertain prognosis.)

J. Has been told that if he does not take it easy, he will have a severe attack.
(Validating factor: No symptoms were given, some functional restriction if the condition is to be controlled.)

K. Has had something which has left him deaf.
(Validating factors: Person had an illness and was left with a permanent handicap, but not as severe for most people as B.)

L. Is recovering but still in bed.
(Validating factors: Person has a functional incapacity, but prognosis is good.)

Before proceeding with our investigation, we should determine whether these factors (legitimization by physician, symptoms, functional incapacity, and prognosis) are, in fact, discriminators in the validation of the status "sick." If those factors are discriminators, there should be some correlation between responses containing the same factors[4] (e.g., two descriptions containing functional incapacities). Therefore, as an initial step in testing whether these factors are discriminators, responses to each of the illness descriptions were cross-correlated. As can be seen in Table 1, descriptions having common elements have a much higher correlation than descriptions lacking common elements.

TABLE 1. *Phi Coefficients for Sick–Not-Sick Matrix**

Description	A	B	C	D	E	F	G	H	I	J	K	L
A. Has pneumonia		.02	.08	.02	.02	.06	.05	.00	.15	.03	.08	.0
B. Lost use of legs			.15	.34	.09	.19	.14	.14	.03	.18	.44	.1
C. Recovering but not working				.30	.12	.16	.30	.13	.14	.13	.20	.3
D. Unable to do strenuous work					.16	.22	.24	.15	.09	.23	.34	.1
E. Stomach pains but can work						.24	.25	.23	.13	.06	.04	.1
F. Arthritis							.23	.43	.22	.15	.18	.1
G. Under doctor's care but can work								.18	.14	.14	.19	.2
H. Rheumatism									.22	.15	.14	.1
I. Controlled illness										.12	.07	.1
J. Will have severe attack with exertion											.22	.0
K. Deaf												.1
L. Bedridden but recovering												

* N = 808. Significance level of correlation is 0.06 at the 1 per cent level.

Upon analyzing the clusters of responses, this relationship became more vivid. Each of the clusters has common elements that are readily identifiable. For instance, Cluster 1 has as its common element a past illness which in some manner limits

[4] Relationship between descriptions on which there is near unanimity of response would not be revealed by this method.

a person's current activity. Both descriptions in Cluster 2 describe chronic illnesses which are associated with pain and impairment. The third cluster contains conditions in which the prognosis is good, but the person is still functionally incapacitated. The final cluster contains conditions which allow the person to continue working.

CLUSTER 1. *Past Illness—Functional Incapacity*

	B	K	D
B. Had something a year ago and as a result lost use of legs.		.44	.34
K. Has had something which has left him deaf.			.34
D. Had something five years ago and since then cannot do strenuous work.			

CLUSTER 2. *Chronic Illness*

	F	H
F. Has had arthritis for past several years.		.43
H. Has increasingly bad attacks of rheumatism.		

CLUSTER 3. *Recovering*

	C	L
C. Is recovering but not yet back to work.		.35
L. Is recovering but still in bed.		

CLUSTER 4. *Ailment Not Interfering with Work*

	E	G
E. Has persistent pains in stomach but can still work.		.25
G. Is under doctor's care but can work.		

Thus, both the intercorrelations and the cluster analysis support the hypothesis that these four factors do act as criteria in legitimatizing the status sick. The manner in which these criteria act as discriminators will be the next concern. Specifically, I will attempt to determine the relative weight of these factors in validating the status sick and whether the importance of these factors varies with socioeconomic status.

When the descriptions are ordered in terms of the percentage of respondents who defined a given condition as sick (Table 2),

TABLE 2. *Per Cent of Persons (N = 808) Who Define a Given Description as Sick or Not Sick*

Description	Sick	Not Sick	Don't Know or No Answer
A. Has pneumonia	95	2	3
I. Illness keeps him in bed on and off	92	4	4
H. Increasingly bad rheumatism	84	13	3.5
E. Persistent pains in stomach, can work	79	18	3
J. Must take it easy	74	22	4
L. Recovering but in bed	73	23	4
F. Has arthritis	70	25.5	4
C. Recovering but not yet back to work	65	32	3
G. Under doctor's care, can work	56	39	5.5
D. Had something five years ago and since then cannot do strenuous work	53.5	43	4
B. Lost use of legs	31.5	65	3
K. Is deaf	24	74	2

it becomes obvious that the percentages vary greatly for the twelve descriptions. For example, 95 per cent of the respondents said that a person who "has a severe case of pneumonia" is sick, while only 24 per cent said that a person who "had something which has left him deaf" is sick.

When the effect of prognosis upon the identification of someone as sick is examined, it is found that the four descriptions most often identified as sick are characterized by an uncertain or worsening prognosis.

CATEGORY 1. *Serious Prognosis*—Uncertain or Worsening

    A.   Has a severe case of pneumonia.

    I.   Has an illness which keeps him in bed on and off. It has gotten worse, and there appears little hope that it will improve.

    H.   Has increasingly bad attacks of rheumatism.

    E.   Has persistent pains in the stomach but can still work.[5]

In the next group, of the four conditions most often defined as sick, three referred to persons in the process of being cured or with a controllable illness.

CATEGORY 2. *Favorable Prognosis*—Controllable or
                  Recovering

    J.   Has been told that if he does not take it easy, he will have a severe attack (controllable).

    L.   Is recovering but still in bed (recovering).

    C.   Is recovering but not yet back to work (recovering).

The descriptions of persons who are physically impaired by a past illness were least often identified as sick.[6]

CATEGORY 3. *Functional Incapacity*—Past Illness

    D.   Had something five years ago and since then cannot do strenuous work.

    B.   Had something a year ago and as a result lost the use of his legs.

    K.   Has had something which has left him deaf.

---

[5] E is considered in this category because the symptomatology may imply a malignancy and hence prognosis is uncertain. However, even if excluded, it would not affect the findings.

[6] Description F (Has had arthritis for the past several years) and Description G (Is under a doctor's care but can work) do not refer to prognosis.

Differences between the three categories are statistically significant at the $p<.01$ level. It is evident, therefore, that when the prognosis is uncertain or worsening, there is a very strong tendency to define a person as sick. The anticipated state of an illness plays a key role in the validation of the status sick.

A not unexpected finding is that persons confined to bed are more often considered sick than persons who are simply unable to work. Thus, when the prognosis is held constant (i.e., analyzed for functional incapacity within a given prognosis group), 92 per cent of the respondents described as sick a person who "has an illness which keeps him in bed on and off," while 79 per cent stated that a person who "has persistent pains in the stomach but can still work" is sick.[7] Similarly, when the conditions in the favorable prognosis category are considered, it is found that 73 per cent of the respondents felt that someone who "is recovering but still in bed" was sick, while 65 per cent said that someone who "is recovering but not yet back to work" was sick.

Description E (Persistent pains in stomach) and Description G (Under doctor's care) were used to explore the differential effect that symptomatology and legitimization by a physician had upon the identification of someone as sick. Both descriptions are similar in that there is no functional incapacity (i.e., a person can work), but they differ in that Description G makes no mention of pain or symptomatology while Description E says nothing of a physician. Seventy-nine per cent of the respondents stated that the person who "has persistent pains in the stomach but can still work" was sick, while only 56 per cent said that the person who "is under a doctor's care but can work" was sick. This finding indicates that, in the absence of functional incapacity, the tendency for a person to be defined as sick is greater if he reports persistent pain than if he reports that he is under a doctor's care.

The initial ordering of the responses to the twelve descriptions, in terms of the percentage who identified a given description as sick, thus reveals the following:

---

[7] All differences mentioned in the text are statistically significant at $p<.01$ unless otherwise noted.

1. The anticipated prognosis or outcome of an illness plays a key, if not a dominant, role in the social identification of someone as sick. The poorer or more uncertain the anticipated consequence, the greater the tendency to define someone as sick.

2. Persons who are physically impaired by a past illness (handicapped) are least often identified as being sick.

3. Persons who are confined to bed are more likely to be defined as sick than persons who cannot work because of an illness.

4. If a person can continue to work, there is a greater tendency to identify him as sick on the basis of persistent pain than on the basis of his being under medical care.

These findings apply to general trends existing in the population of New York City. However, as I have indicated, there may be multimodal response patterns. Consequently, the over-all patterning of responses to these descriptions may cover up, rather than reflect, the response patterns of different social groups. Since socioeconomic status has frequently been related to variations in attitude, the responses were further analyzed in terms of socioeconomic factors—specifically, by the main wage-earners' income and by the respondents' education. The respondents were divided into three income groups (under $4,000, $4,000–$7,499, $7,500 and over) and three education groups (8 years or less of schooling, or grade school; 9–12 years, or high school; more than 12 years, or college).[8]

When the descriptions are ordered in terms of the percentage of persons who define a given condition as sick, there are only minor differences among the three income groups (Table 3). However, when we examine the percentage of persons who define a given description as sick, interesting differences emerge. In the case of the descriptions in Category 1 (Serious Prognosis),

[8] The terms grade school, high school, and college will be used for the respective categories of years of schooling. Whatever discrepancies occur between these categories and years of schooling (e.g., some persons in the grade school group having no schooling) will be negligible.

TABLE 3. *Rank Order of Descriptions in Terms of Per Cent of Persons in the Low, Middle, or High-Income Group Defining a Description as Sick*

Descriptions as Ranked by Total Population	Total Population (N=808)		Low-Income Group (N=272)		Middle-Income Group (N=327)		High-Income Group (N=108)	
	Rank	Per Cent	Rank	Per Cent	Rank	Per Cent	Rank	Per Cent
Group 1								
A. Has pneumonia	1	96	1	95	1	99	1	100
I. Illness keeps him in bed on and off	2	92	2	90	2	94	2	94
H. Increasingly bad rheumatism	3	84	3	82.5	3	85	3	82
E. Persistent pains in stomach, can work	4	79	4	77	4	78.9	4	79.5
Group 2								
J. Must take it easy	5	74	5	76	5	78.7	6	59.5
L. Recovering, but in bed	6	73	7	73.2	6	75	5	67
F. Has arthritis	7	70	6	73.9	7	69.5	7	59
C. Recovering, but not back to work	8	65	8	66	8	68	8	57
G. Under a doctor's care, but can work	9	56	9	64	9	55	9	42
Group 3								
D. Had something five years ago and since then cannot do strenuous work	10	53.5	10	57	10	53	10	38
B. Lost use of legs	11	31.5	11	40	11	26	11	20.5
K. Is deaf	12	24	12	34	12	18	12	7

TABLE 4. *Per Cent of Persons in Each Income Group Who Define a Given Description in Category 1 (Serious Prognosis) as Sick*

Description	Under $4,000 (N=272)	$4,000– $7,499 (N=327)	$7,500 and Over (N=108)
A. Has pneumonia	95	99	100
I. Illness keeps him in bed on and off	90	94	94
H. Increasingly bad rheumatism	82.5	85	82
E. Persistent pains in stomach, can work	77	79	79.5
Mean	*86*	*89*	*89*

there were slight and statistically non-significant differences between the three income groups (Table 4). Almost all respondents defined these conditions as sick.

On the other hand, larger percentages in the lower- and middle-income groups than in the upper-income groups defined the Category 2 descriptions (Favorable Prognosis) as sick (Table 5).

The mean percentage of respondents who defined the three descriptions as sick in the upper group is 61, while for the middle-income group it is 74 and for the lower-income group is 72. The

TABLE 5. *Per Cent of Persons in Each Income Group Who Define a Given Description in Category 2 (Favorable Prognosis) as Sick*

Description	Under $4,000 (N=272)	$4,000– $7,499 (N=327)	$7,500 and Over (N=108)
J. Must take it easy	76	79	59.5
L. Recovering but in bed	73	75	67
C. Recovering but not back to work	66	68	57
Mean	*72*	*74*	*61*

difference between the lower- and the upper-income groups is significant at $p<.05$, while the difference between the middle- and the upper-income groups is significant at $p<.01$.

For the three descriptions of Category 3 (Functional Incapacity), the upper-income group has the lowest per cent of sick responses and the middle-income group falls between the upper- and the lower-income groups. The mean percentage of persons who defined the descriptions in Category 3 as sick is 22 in the upper-income group, 32 in the middle-income group, and 44 in the lower-income group (Table 6). The difference

TABLE 6. *Per Cent of Persons in Each Income Group Who Define a Given Description in Category 3 (Functional Incapacity) as Sick*

Description	Under $4,000 (N=272)	$4,000– $7,499 (N=327)	$7,500 and Over (N=108)
D. Had something five years ago and since then cannot do strenuous work	57	53	38
B. Lost use of legs	40	26	20.5
K. Is deaf	34	18	7
Mean	*44*	*32*	*22*

between the lower- and the upper-income groups is significant at $p<.01$, while the difference between the middle- and the upper-income groups is significant at $p<.05$.

Respondents in each of the three income groups defined the Serious Prognosis descriptions as sick much more often than they did the descriptions in either Category 2 (Favorable Prognosis) or Category 3 (Incapacity) and the descriptions in Category 3 were least often defined as sick (Table 7). Thus, within each income group, the poorer or more uncertain the prognosis, the greater the tendency to define a condition as sick.

These findings lead to the conclusion that if a person has an illness with an uncertain or worsening prognosis, a greater percentage of persons in all income groups will tend to define him as sick than will define a person who is more incapacitated but

TABLE 7. *Mean Per Cent of Sick Responses in Each Income Group to Each Anticipated Consequences Category**

Consequences Category	Under $4,000 (N=272)	$4,000– $7,499 (N=327)	$7,500 and Over (N=108)
Category 1 Serious Prognosis—	86	89	89
Category 2 Favorable Prognosis—	72	74	61
Category 3 Functional Incapacity—	44	32	22

* Within each income group, all differences between the anticipated consequences categories are significant at $p < .01$.

has a good prognosis. Indeed, when the responses to specific descriptions are examined, it is found that Description I (partially bedridden, a poor prognosis) was defined as sick much more often than Description L (totally bedridden, a favorable prognosis) (Table 8).

TABLE 8. *Per Cent of Sick Responses in Each Income Group to Description I and Description L**

Description	Under $4,000 (N=272)	$4,000– $7,499 (N=327)	$7,500 and Over (N=108)
I. Has an illness which keeps him in bed on and off. It has gotten worse, and there appears little hope it will improve.	90	94	94
L. Is recovering but still in bed.	73	75	67

* All differences between Descriptions I and L are significant at $p < .01$.

Table 7, however, also shows an inverse relationship between income and the tendency to define conditions falling into Category 2 and Category 3 as sick. It is found, for example, that the percentage of persons in the low-income group who defined incapacitating conditions as sick (44 per cent) was twice as large as the corresponding percentage (22) of persons in the upper-income group. This difference is significant at $p<.01$. Since each description in Category 3 refers to a condition with a known non-fatal prognosis and a functional incapacity, the differences in response indicate a greater tendency on the part of respondents in the low-income group to consider functional incapacity in and of itself as a valid criterion for defining someone as sick.

This tendency in the low-income group is further substantiated by the responses to Description H (Has increasingly bad attacks of rheumatism) and Description F (Has had arthritis for the past several years). The illnesses mentioned in both descriptions are commonly associated with both chronicity and functional incapacities and are so similar in terms of symptoms, limitations upon activity, and prognosis that they are often confused in the layman's mind. One description, however, refers to a worsening prognosis (Increasingly bad attacks of rheumatism), while the other makes no mention of the prognosis (Has had arthritis for the past several years).

Table 9 shows no difference between the upper- and the lower-income groups in response to the worsening condition (Descrip-

TABLE 9. *Per Cent of Sick Responses in Each Income Group to Description F and Description H**

Description	Under $4,000 (N=272)	$4,000– $7,499 (N=327)	$7,500 and Over (N=108)
F. Has had arthritis for the past several years	73	69.5	59
H. Has increasingly bad attacks of rheumatism	82.5	85	82

* All differences between Descriptions F and H are significant at $p<.01$.

tion H). There is, however, a large difference between the response of these two groups when there is no mention of prognosis (Description E). Seventy-three per cent of the persons in the low-income group and only 59 per cent in the upper-income group defined Description F as sick. Thus, when a description implies both functional incapacity and worsening prognosis, there is no significant difference in response patterns between the upper- and the lower-income groups. However, when a description implies only the existence of functional incapacity, significantly larger percentages of respondents in the low-income group will define the description as sick ($p<.01$). Since the symptomatology of these two conditions is both similar and severe, this finding also strongly supports the position that prognosis is more important than symptomatology as a criterion in the validation of the status sick.

It appears, therefore, that for all income groups, the prognosis is a more important factor than functional incapacity in validation of the status "sick." But the magnitude of the difference between these two factors decreases as income decreases.

The importance of being under a doctor's care as a criterion in the validation of the status sick varies inversely with income. For instance, 64 per cent in the low income, 55 per cent in the middle income, and 42 per cent in the upper-income groups defined as sick someone who is under a doctor's care but can work (Description G). The differences between the low-income group and the middle- or the upper-income group are significant at $p<.05$.

Responses were also analyzed in terms of the respondents' education in order to investigate in more detail the effect that factors associated with socioeconomic status have upon the criteria for the status sick. Response patterns of low-income and grade school, or middle-income and high school, or high-income and college groups were affected selectively in a given direction by either income or education. As can be seen in Table 10, there is great similarity between responses analyzed in terms of income and those analyzed in terms of education. Two interesting sets of differences are found though for the most part they are not statistically significant.

TABLE 10. *Per Cent of Sick Responses in Each Income and Education Group to a Given Description*

Description	Grade School Education (N=240)	Low Income (N=272)	High School Education (N=392)	Middle Income (N=327)	College Education (N=163)	High Income (N=108)
Group 1						
A. Has pneumonia	95	95	98.5	99	100	100
I. Illness keeps him in bed on and off	89	90	93	94	93	94
H. Increasingly bad rheumatism	82	82.5	84	85	87	82
E. Persistent pains in stomach, can work	77	77	79.5	79	79	79.5
Group 2						
J. Must take it easy	77	76	78	79	59	59.5
L. Recovering but in bed	77	73	69	75	78	67*
F. Has had arthritis for past several years	76	73	70	69.5	62	59
C. Recovering but not yet back to work	67	66	63	68	66	57
G. Under a doctor's care but can work	63	64	52	55	52	42
Group 3						
D. Had something five years ago and since then cannot do strenuous work	63	57	54	53	37	38
B. Lost use of legs	45	40	29	26	15	20.5
K. Is deaf	39	34	19	18	11	7

* This difference between the high-education group and the high-income group in response to Description L was the only difference that approached significance ($p<.05$).

TABLE 11. *Per Cent of Sick Responses in Grade School and Low-Income Groups to Descriptions D, B, and K*

Description	Grade School Education (N=240)	Income under $4,000 (N=272)	Significance of Difference Between Income and Education Groups
D. Had something five years ago and since then cannot do strenuous work	63	57	N.S.*
B. Lost use of legs	45	40	N.S.
K. Is deaf	39	34	N.S.

* N.S. = non-significant.

1. When the low-income group is compared with the grade school group, it is found that the grade school group has larger percentages of sick responses to all items in the Functional Incapacity Category than has the low-income group (Table 11).

2. When the high-income group is compared with the college group, it is found that the college group has larger percentages of sick responses to three of the conditions in the Favorable Prognosis Category than does the high-income group (Table 12).

A possible explanation for these differences is that the low-income group contains more status-mobile, young respondents, whose reference group is higher and whose potential resources

TABLE 12. *Per Cent of Sick Responses in College and High-Income Groups to Descriptions C and L*

Description	College Education (N=163)	Income $7,500 and Over (N=108)	Significance of Difference Between Income and Education Groups
C. Recovering but not yet back to work	66	57	N.S.*
L. Recovering but in bed	78	67	.05

* N.S. = non-significant.

are greater than their income indicates. The differences between the high-income and the college groups also appear attributable to the existence of status-mobile persons. However, in this instance it is the educational group that contains the greater number of status-mobile persons. In the college group, the status-mobile persons, using education as a primary means of upward mobility, have a lower reference group and less resources than their education indicates. If this reasoning is correct, then the response pattern of non-mobile persons in the low socioeconomic groups (e.g., persons with low income and grade school education) would be more similar to the grade school group than to the low-income group. Similarly, the response pattern of non-mobile persons in the high socioeconomic group (e.g., persons with high income and college education) would be more similar to the high-income group than to the college group. Indeed, as Table 13 shows, the response pattern of persons in the low-

TABLE 13. *Per Cent of Sick Responses in Low-Income, Grade School, and Low-Income–Grade School Groups to Descriptions D, B, and K*

Description	Low Income (N=272)	Grade School Education (N=240)	Low-Income– Grade School Education (N=122)
D. Had something five years ago and since then cannot do strenuous work	57	63	64.5
B. Lost use of legs	40	45	48
K. Is deaf	34	39	45

income–low-education group is closer to the pattern of the grade school group than to that of the low-income group. Furthermore, Table 14 shows that the response pattern of the high-income–college group is closer to the pattern of the high-income group than to that of the college group.

It should be noted that only two differences in Tables 13 and 14 approach significance ($p<.05$), namely, the difference between the low-income–grade school group and the low-income

TABLE 14. *Per Cent of Sick Responses in High-Income, College, and High-Income–College Groups to Descriptions C, L, and G*

Description	High Income (N=108)	College Education (N=163)	High-Income– College Education (N=61)
C. Recovering but not yet back to work	57	66	57
L. Recovering but in bed	67	78	69
G. Under a doctor's care but can work	42	52	41

group in response to Description K, and the difference between the high-income and college groups in response to Description L. Thus, whether the observed differences between these income and education groups reflect true population parameters is questionable.

But even if these differences do reflect true population parameters, the differences seem to relate to status mobility rather than to the differential effect of income or education. Analysis of the responses of those persons who fall into the low-income–grade school groups and those persons who fall into the high-income–college group provide insight into the over-all effect of socioeconomic status on illness attitudes.[9]

The tendency to use either incapacity or prognosis as the basis for defining someone as sick is somewhat greater in the low-status group than in either the low-income or the grade school groups. For example, the average percentage of persons defining the conditions in the incapacitated category (3) as sick is 53 in the low-status group, 44 in the low-income group, and 49 in the grade school group. The difference between the low-status group and the low-income group is significant at $p<.05$. Furthermore, the low-status group is the only analytic group studied in which the difference in the percentage of sick

[9] For clarity, the low-income, grade school education group will be referred to as the low socioeconomic status or low-status group and the high-income, college group will be referred to as the high socioeconomic status or high-status group.

TABLE 15. *Per Cent of Persons in Low-Income–Grade School Group (N=122) Who Defined Descriptions H, F, C, and D as Sick or Not Sick*

Description	Sick	Not Sick	Don't Know
H. Has increasingly bad attacks of rheumatism	81.5	11	7
F. Has had arthritis for past several years	79	14	7
C. Recovering but not yet back to work	63	28	9
D. Had something five years ago and since then cannot do strenuous work	64.5	26	10

responses between Description H and Description F or between Description C and Description D is under 3 per cent (Table 15).

On the other hand, though statistically non-significant, the tendency to disregard function as a factor in defining a person as sick is consistently found to be somewhat greater in the high-status group than in either the high-income or the college group. For example, the average percentage of persons defining the incapacitating conditions as sick is 19 in the high-status group, 22 in the high-income group, and 21 in the college group. Moreover, the difference between the percentages of persons

TABLE 16. *Per Cent of Sick Responses in High-Income, College, and High-Income–College Groups to Descriptions H and F*

Description	High Income (N=108)	College Education (N=163)	High-Income– College Education (N=61)
H. Has increasingly bad attacks of rheumatism	82	87	86
F. Has had arthritis for past several years	59	62	55
Difference	23	25	31

who defined Description H and Description F as sick is greater in the high-status group than in either the high-income or the college groups (Table 16).

Consequently, a comparison of the high-status and low-status groups substantiates still further the conclusions about prognosis and function which result from the income and education analysis. Table 17 shows, for example, that the mean percentage

TABLE 17. *Per Cent of Persons in the Low-Status and High-Status Groups Who Defined Given Descriptions in Category 3 (Functional Incapacity) as Sick*

Description	Low Status (N=122)	High Status (N=61)	Significance of Difference between Groups
			$p<$
D. Had something five years ago and since then cannot do strenuous work	63	32	.01
B. Had something a year ago and as a result lost the use of his legs	48	16	.01
K. Has had something which has left him deaf	45	8.5	.01
Mean	*52*	*19*	*.01*

of persons in the low-status group who defined the conditions in Category 3 as sick is almost three times as large as the corresponding percentage in the high-status group.

Similarly the mean percentage of persons defining the descriptions in Category 2 (Favorable Prognosis) as sick is 70 in the low-status group and 59 in the high-status group. The difference in these percentages is significant at $p<.01$. Further pointing up the over-all importance of prognosis as a factor in the validation of the status sick is the fact that well over 80 per cent of the respondents in both the high- and low-status groups defined the descriptions in Category 1 (Serious Prognosis) as sick (Table 18).

The comparison of the high- and low-status groups also shows an inverse relationship between socioeconomic status and the tendency to define someone as sick because he is under a doctor's

TABLE 18. *Mean Per Cent of Sick Responses in the Low-Status and High-Status Groups to Each Anticipated Consequences Category*

Category	Low Status (N=122)	High Status (N=61)	Significance of Difference Between Groups
1. Serious Prognosis	84.5	88	N.S.
2. Favorable Prognosis	70	59	$p<.01$
3. Functional Incapacity	52	19	$p<.01$

care. It was found that while 63 per cent of the persons in the low-status group defined Description G (Is under a doctor's care, but can work) as sick, only 4 per cent in the high-status group did so. This difference is significant at $p<.01$.

Consequently the findings resulting from the comparison of the low and high socioeconomic groups as well as the findings resulting from the income and education analysis, support the following hypotheses:

> *Hypothesis 1.* There is an inverse relationship between socioeconomic status and the importance of functional or physical incapacity as a factor in identifying someone as sick.
>
> *Hypothesis 3.* The poorer or more uncertain the prognosis, the greater the tendency to define someone as sick.

On the basis of the same findings the following hypothesis can be rejected:

> *Hypothesis 2.* In the absence of physical and functional incapacity, there is a direct relationship between socioeconomic status and the tendency to define someone as sick on the basis of his being under a physician's care.

The relationship between socioeconomic status and the tendency to define someone as sick on the basis of his being under a doctor's care is inverse rather than direct.

Furthermore, of the factors studied (functional incapacity, medical attention, prognosis and symptomatology) the most important single factor for all socioeconomic groups in the validation of the status sick is prognosis.

Chapter Five

Behavioral Expectations Relevant to Illness

Behavioral Expectations Regarding an Ill Person

The findings of Chapter IV bring into question the assumption of a unimodal sick role. If validating criteria vary systematically, should we not also expect systematic variations in behavioral expectations? In examining this and other questions relevant to the expectations associated with illness, I have followed Parsons' lead and concentrated on those areas he feels are relevant to the sick role: (1) expectations regarding social responsibility; (2) expectations regarding patient care, including information and physical comfort; and (3) expectations regarding technically competent help.

Inherent in any discussion of the sick role is the recognition that the behaviors of both the sick person and the significant others in his environment are legitimate only insofar as they are aimed at getting the sick person well. Parsons, for instance, states:

> The third element is the definition of the state of being ill as itself undesirable with its obligation to want to "get well." The first two elements of legitimation of the sick role thus are conditional in a highly important sense. It is a

71

relative legitimation so long as he is in this unfortunate state which both he and alter hope he can get out of as expeditiously as possible.[1]

Given the functional nexus of the statuses associated with illness, it seems likely that role expectations would be determined to some extent by the prognosis or anticipated consequences of an illness. Thus, behaviors which might be appropriate when an illness has a poor prognosis may very well be inappropriate when an illness has a good prognosis. Specifically, in terms of the behavioral areas referred to above it was hypothesized that, as the prognosis varies from controlled and known to unknown and serious, the tendency increases to treat the ill person as dependent, or in Parsons' usage as "sick."

To test this and other hypotheses, the respondents were given the following descriptions of illness states:

a) a person's illness appears to be getting worse.

b) a person appears to be getting better.

c) the illness is critical.

d) a person is suffering from a chronic illness (arthritis, rheumatism) or from the permanent effects of an illness (lameness).

e) a person complains over a period of time that he isn't feeling well (has aches or nausea or discomfort), can still work, but doesn't know why he isn't feeling up to par.

f) a person has an illness, such as diabetes, and can go about his daily routines so long as he follows his doctor's orders and takes the right medicine.

The respondents were then asked to select from each of the following four lists what they felt was the best thing to do when a person had each of the conditions described above:

List A. Medical Care

1. See to it that he sees a doctor.

[1] Talcott Parsons, *The Social System* (Glencoe, Ill.: Free Press, 1951), p. 437.

2. Encourage him to see a doctor.
3. Discourage him from running to a doctor with small aches and pains.
4. See to it that he doesn't run to a doctor with small aches and pains.

List B. Physical Comfort
1. Give him a great deal of extra care.
2. See to it that he is comfortable.
3. Encourage him to do things for himself.
4. Treat him like everybody else.

List C. Social Responsibility
1. Make major decisions for him.
2. Keep responsibilities and worries from him.
3. Encourage him to do some sort of work.
4. Urge him to carry his daily responsibilities.

List D. Information
1. Make sure that he tells you about any changes in his condition no matter how unimportant they seem.
2. Discourage him from bothering you about every little ache and pain.
3. Encourage him to tell you about any changes in his condition no matter how unimportant they seem.
4. Steer him away from bothering you about every little ache and pain.

As one moves down a given list from statement 1 to statement 4, the tendency increases to treat the ill person as non-dependent (1 = maximum dependence, 4 = maximum independence).

If the hypothesis regarding prognosis is correct, it would be expected that as these conditions increase in seriousness[2] and uncertainty the behavioral expectations associated with a condition would be increasingly dependent and, as a consequence, the following should occur:

[2] "Seriousness" refers to danger of loss of life.

	Condition	Prognosis	Expected Result
c)	Critical	Very serious, extremely uncertain	Highest dependency
a)	Worse	Worsening, uncertain	
e)	Not up to par	Apparently non-serious, unknown rather than uncertain	
b)	Better	Non-serious, apparently known	
f)	Controlled	Non-serious, known	Lowest dependency

As can be seen from Table 19, the findings verify the hypothesis that, as the prognosis becomes more serious and uncertain, the tendency increases to treat an ill person as dependent.

In the prediction of response to Condition d (chronic illness or permanent handicap) was excluded because the analysis of the criteria validating the status sick indicates that it contains two separate elements, each of which evokes a somewhat different response.[3] These two are arthritis, which is chronic and may get worse, and lameness, which has a known prognosis. Neverthe-

TABLE 19. *Tendency to Treat Ill Person as Dependent*

	Condition	Prognosis	Mean Response to Lists A, B, C, D*
c)	Critical	Very serious, extremely uncertain	1.42†
a)	Worse	Worsening, uncertain	1.68
e)	Not up to par	Apparently non-serious, unknown rather than uncertain	2.46
b)	Better	Non-serious, apparently known	2.68
f)	Controlled	Non-serious, known	2.90

* The higher the mean the higher the dependency.
† All differences between conditions are significant at $p < .01$.

[3] See discussion in Chapter IV.

less, since both arthritis and lameness involve severe physical and functional incapacity, the responses to Condition d enable us to compare the importance of prognosis and of functional or physical incapacity as factors in determining the extent to which a person will be treated as dependent.

If the respondents tend to treat a person as sick or dependent primarily in terms of the extent of his incapacity, it would be expected that illnesses encompassed by Condition d would elicit more responses than would conditions which do not have, or do not refer to, functional and physical incapacity. The contrary is found. For example, the mean responses to Condition d and to Condition e, which specifically refers to mild discomforts, are identical—2.46. Furthermore, as shown in Table 20,

TABLE 20. *Tendency to Treat Ill Person as Dependent*
When He Has Condition a, c, *or* d

Condition		Mean Responses To Lists A, B, C, D*
d)	Chronic	2.46
c)	Critical	1.42
a)	Worse	1.68

* Differences between Condition c or a and Condition d are significant at $p<.01$.

when the responses to Condition d are compared with the responses to Condition c (Critical) and Condition a (Worse), neither of which refers to incapacities, it is found that the tendency to treat the ill person as dependent is very much stronger in the responses to Conditions c and a than in the responses to Condition d.

Given the fact that responses to a condition with serious physical and functional incapacity and to a condition with minor physical and functional incapacity are similar and that the tendency to treat the ill person as dependent is much greater with respect to Conditions c and a than with respect to Condition d, the behaviors which Parsons postulates as being associated with the sick role appear determined to a greater extent by prognosis than by (the presence of) functional and physical incapacity.

Given the fact that there is variation in response to prognosis, the question remains: Do the responses to the various conditions represent a single statistical dimension, or do they represent entirely different statistical dimensions?[4] In other words, do the responses to a given prognosis enable one to predict the response to another prognosis?

This problem is crucial because the assumption that responses are scalable or continuous is inherent in the work of Parsons, Mechanic, and Apple. That is, as a person displays more signs of illness, he is progressively treated as dependent. Parsons states, for example: "First, it must be remembered that there is an enormous range of different types of illness, and of degrees of severity. Hence a certain abstraction is inevitable in any such general account as the present one."[5] However, it is quite possible that the behavioral expectations towards illness are neither continuous nor scalable.

In order to determine the extent to which responses to the various conditions reflect a single statistical dimension, the responses were cluster analyzed. This analysis revealed the following two clusters:

CLUSTER 5

		a	c
a)	Illness getting worse	—	.32
c)	Illness critical		—

CLUSTER 6

		e	f	d	b
e)	Not up to par	—	.30	.43	.35
f)	Illness controlled		—	.40	.43
d)	Illness chronic			—	.45
b)	Illness better				—

[4] Of course, this question is pertinent only so long as a person remains able to function to some extent. If a person is physically helpless, he must be treated as a dependent if he is to survive.

[5] Parsons, *op. cit.*, p. 440.

Not only do two clusters emerge, but an examination of Table 21 reveals that the correlation between the responses to the conditions in Cluster 5 and the conditions in Cluster 6 is negligible. Furthermore, three of the eight possible correlations between responses to the conditions in Clusters 5 and 6 are negative.

Consequently, there appear to be two distinct and unrelated sets of behavioral expectations relevant to the ill person. The behavioral expectations reflected in Cluster 5 occur when prognosis is serious and uncertain. On the other hand, those expectancies reflected in Cluster 6 occur when health is impaired but the prognosis appears non-serious. In order to distinguish the two sets of behavioral expectations, the first will be referred to as the "sick role" and the second as the "impaired role."

To distinguish clearly between the sick role and the impaired role, it is necessary to examine in some detail the response pattern within each cluster. For each of the behavior areas studied, Table 22 indicates a significant difference between responses to the conditions in the fifth and the sixth clusters.

The responses elicited by the conditions in Cluster 5 reflect a consistent tendency to treat the ill person as dependent or sick. On the other hand, the responses elicited by the conditions in Cluster 6 reflect a tendency to encourage the ill person to be independent in regard to personal care and social responsibility and at the same time a tendency to encourage him to seek medical care.

TABLE 21. *Correlation Coefficients for Responses to Illness Conditions*

Condition	a	b	c	d	e	f
a) Worse	—	(.08)	.32	(.04)	(.18)	(.03)
b) Better		—	(−.05)	.26	.35	.43
c) Critical			—	(−.05)	(.06)	(−.14)
d) Chronic				—	.25	.40
e) Not up to par					—	.30
f) Controlled						—

Figures in parentheses refer to correlations between responses to conditions in Clusters 5 and 6.

TABLE 22. *Central Tendency of Responses to Conditions in Cluster 5 (Sick) and Cluster 6 (Impaired) for Each of the Four Types of Behavior**

Behavior	Mean	CLUSTER 5 Tendency	Mean	CLUSTER 6 Tendency
Medical care	1.49	*Between:* See to it he sees a doctor, *and* Encourage him to see a doctor.	2.28	Encourage him to see a doctor.
Physical Comfort	1.41	Give them a great deal of extra care.	2.72	Encourage them to do things for themselves.
Social Responsibility	1.89	Keep responsibilities and worries away from them.	3.02	Encourage them to do some sort of useful work.
Information	1.59	*Between:* Make sure they tell you about any changes in their condition, *and* Encourage them to tell you about any changes in their condition.	2.50	*Between:* Encourage them to tell you about any changes in their condition, *and* Discourage them from bothering you about every ache and pain.

* All differences between responses to Cluster 5 and Cluster 6 are significant at $p < .01$.

This is not meant to imply that, in regard to physical care and social responsibility, there are no differences in the behaviors associated with the impaired role and the healthy role. Quite the contrary. Within Cluster 6 the central tendency in the areas of self-responsibility and personal care is the third item in each list ("Encourage them to do things for themselves" and "Encourage them to do some sort of useful work") rather than the fourth item ("Urge them to carry their daily responsibilities" and "Treat them like everybody else"). Furthermore, there is a tendency to seek additional knowledge, which could in turn lead to a redefinition of the ill person's role. These findings imply that there is recognition of the impairment caused by the conditions in Cluster 6 and that extra effort is involved if the impaired person is to be independent.

The supportive behavior associated with what I have termed the "impaired role" is, on the basis of the evidence, distinctly different from, and not related to, the behaviors associated with the "sick role." In the case of the impaired role, the social pressure serves to aid and maintain normal behavior within the limitations of a given condition, while in the case of the sick role, the social pressure serves to discourage normal behavior. Therefore, in terms of function, the two roles are opposites, and it is clear why there is little correlation between behavioral expectations in Cluster 5 and Cluster 6.

Turning to the question of consensus it is found that there is greater agreement on how to behave when conditions in Cluster 5 occur than when conditions in Cluster 6 occur (Table 23).[6]

The question which arises is: Does the relatively high variation in responses to the conditions in Cluster 6 result from a general lack of consensus throughout the population, or does it reflect socioeconomic variations? Referring to the work of Koos[7]

[6] The relatively high variance of Condition *d*, as shown in Table 23, further supports my feeling that this condition contains two discrete elements. Variance of Condition *d* is significantly greater than other conditions at $p<.01$.

[7] Earl Lomon Koos, "Illness in Regionville," in Dorrian Apple (ed.), *Studies of Health and Sickness* (New York: McGraw Hill Book Co., 1960), pp. 7-14.

TABLE 23. *Analysis of Variance of Responses (N=808) to Illness Conditions*

Condition	Variance	Significance of Difference Between Condition a and the Other Conditions	Significance of Difference Between Condition c and the Other Conditions
Cluster 5 (sick)		$p<$	$p<$
c) Critical	.49	—	.05
a) Worse	.55	.05	—
Cluster 6 (impaired)			
b) Better	1.15	.01	.01
e) Not up to par	1.33	.01	.01
f) Controlled	1.37	.01	.01
d) Chronic	1.61	.01	.01

and Saunders,[8] I have reasoned that, since illness of any sort is a more serious economic threat to persons with low incomes than to persons with high incomes, persons with low incomes would have a greater tendency to treat someone as sick in terms of functional impairment than would persons with high income. In addition, persons with limited economic means may find it simpler and easier to treat someone with a condition in Cluster 6 as dependent than to provide the support and resources necessary to encourage independence. Allison Davis, for instance, in his comparison of middle-class and lower-class practices in child-rearing, presents evidence that it may be economically more feasible to treat someone as dependent than to encourage independence. He reports that middle-class parents spend much time and effort training their children to be independent within the home, while lower-class parents, either because both parents work or because there is an absence of labor-saving appliances, lack the time to train and encourage their children and, therefore, treat them as dependent.[9] It was therefore hypothesized that,

[8] Lyle Saunders, *Cultural Differences and Medical Care* (New York: Russell Sage Foundation, 1954).

[9] Allison Davis, "Social Class and Color Differences in Child Rearing," in G. E. Swanson, T. M. Newcomb, and E. L. Hartley (eds.) *Readings in Social Psychology* (New York: Henry Holt and Co., 1952), pp. 539-44.

as socioeconomic status decreased, the tendency increases to treat persons with illnesses that have a non-serious prognosis as sick. To test this hypothesis, the responses to the various conditions were analyzed in terms of income and education. For this analysis, the population was divided into the same income and education groups as those used in Chapter IV.

The response patterns, in terms of the main wage-earner's income, show that in all income groups the tendency to treat an ill person as dependent increases as the prognosis becomes more serious and unknown. As can be seen in Table 24, when responses

TABLE 24. *Mean Response by Low-, Middle-, and High-Income Groups for Each Condition**

Condition	Low Income (N=272)	Middle Income (N=327)	High Income (N=108)
Cluster 5 (Sick)			
c) Critical	1.57	1.43	1.34
a) Worse	1.75	1.67	1.68
Cluster 6 (Impaired)			
e) Not up to par	2.42	2.50	2.51
b) Better	2.59	2.72	2.82
f) Controlled	2.81	3.01	3.10
d) Chronic	2.47	2.51	2.65

* Except for the differences between Conditions d and e, all differences between conditions in a given income group are significant at $p < .01$.

to the various conditions are ordered in terms of the tendency to treat the sick person as dependent, there is no difference between the ordering within any given income group and the ordering for the total population.[10]

Interesting differences between the income groups emerge, however, in the mean responses to each condition. As can be seen in Table 25, there are no significant differences in response between the middle- and the low-income groups in regard to the four conditions in Cluster 6. On the other hand, not only are

[10] See Table 19.

TABLE 25. Significance of Difference in Mean Responses of Low-, Middle-, and High-Income Groups for Each Illness Condition

Condition	Low vs. Middle $p<$	Group with Most Dependency	Low vs. High $p<$	Group with Most Dependency	Middle vs. High $p<$	Group with Most Dependency
Cluster 5 (Sick)						
c) Critical	.01	Middle	.01	High	N.S.	High
a) Worse	N.S.	Middle	N.S.	High	N.S.	Middle
Cluster 6 (Impaired)						
e) Not up to par	N.S.	Low	N.S.	Low	N.S.	Middle
b) Better	N.S.	No Difference	.01	Low	.01	Middle
f) Controlled	N.S.	Low	.01	Low	.01	Middle
d) Chronic	N.S.	Middle	.01	Low	.01	Middle

three of the four differences between the low- and the high-income groups significant at $p<.01$, but in regard to all four conditions, the low-income group treated the ill person as more dependent than did the upper-income group. Similarly, when the responses of the middle- and the high-income groups are compared, it is found that, for all four conditions in Cluster 6, the middle-income group treated the ill person as more dependent than did the upper-income group. The differences between the middle- and the upper-income groups are also significant at $p<.01$ in three of the four instances. Surprisingly, when the responses to the conditions in Cluster 5 (Critical *and* Worse) are examined, it is found that, while there is no significant difference in the responses of the three income groups to Condition *a* (Worse), both the high- and the middle-income groups tend to treat persons with a critical illness as more dependent than do persons in the low-income group ($p<.01$).

In order to determine whether this difference between the high- and the low-income groups might be the result of a large difference in response to a specific behavioral area, the responses to Lists A, B, C, and D were compared. As can be seen in Table 26, in every behavioral area the high-income group treats the person with a critical illness as more dependent than does the low-income group. The fact that this difference between the income groups is consistent throughout all four behavioral areas indicates that there is a basic attitudinal difference between low- and high-income groups in terms of the treatment of the critically ill person.

My feeling is that this occurs because the lower-income group lacks the resources to support extensive dependency. This may seem a contradiction to the earlier hypothesis in regard to Cluster 6. However, I am suggesting that in regard to resource expenditure and dependency the following curvilinear relationship exists: a great deal of time and attention are required for either extensive supportive behavior (maintenance of independency) or extensive care (extreme dependency) while less time and energy are expended on custodial care. If this is true then the low-income groups are not in a position to offer full supportive care either in extreme illness or in rehabilitative situations.

TABLE 26. *Mean Response of Low-, Middle-, and High-Income Groups to Each Illness Condition in Each Behavioral Area*

Behavioral Area and Income Group	Critical	Worse	Not up to Par	Better	Controllable	Chronic
A. Medical Care						
Low income	1.40	1.72	1.94	2.48	2.58	2.17
Middle income	1.29	1.62	1.97	2.49	2.71	2.05
High income	1.24	1.59	1.81	2.66	2.76	2.18
B. Physical Comfort						
Low income	1.43	1.42	2.55	2.65	2.90	2.43
Middle income	1.35	1.46	2.69	2.81	3.27	2.48
High income	1.29	1.49	2.72	2.75	3.28	2.57
C. Social Responsibility						
Low income	1.83	2.08	2.77	2.84	3.27	2.78
Middle income	1.66	2.05	2.90	3.10	3.46	2.99
High income	1.60	2.04	3.05	3.10	3.47	3.13
D. Information						
Low income	1.62	1.81	2.45	2.41	2.51	2.50
Middle income	1.45	1.55	2.45	2.50	2.63	2.55
High income	1.26	1.61	2.49	2.79	2.90	2.82

In the four behavioral areas the pattern for the population as a whole is repeated in each of the income groups (see Table 26). That is, for all conditions, there is: (1) a consistent tendency among all income groups to treat the ill person as most dependent in the area of Medical Care, and least dependent in the area of Social Responsibility; (2) for all income groups within each behavioral area, the tendency to treat an ill person as dependent is directly related to the uncertainty and seriousness of his prognosis; and (3) for all income groups within each behavioral area, there is large and significant difference between the responses to the conditions in Cluster 5 and in Cluster 6. In addition, in no instance do respondents in one income group tend to feel strongly that the proper way to treat a person with a given condition is to encourage dependency while respondents in another income group tend to feel strongly that the proper way to treat a person with that condition is to encourage independency. Thus, as hypothesized, the lower-income groups tend to treat persons with conditions in Cluster 6 as dependent to a greater extent than do the upper-income groups, but this difference is quantitative rather than qualitative.

To investigate in more detail the effect of factors associated with socioeconomic status upon behavioral expectations, responses were also analyzed in terms of the respondents' education. Differences in response between analogous income and education groups would indicate the separate effects of income and education upon responses to the various illness states. Thus the responses of the low-income group were compared with the grade-school group, the middle-income group with the high-school group and the high-income with the college group. Table 27 indicates, however, that with one exception, the differences in response between these groups are negligible and nonsignificant. A further indication of the similarity in response between the income and the education groups is that the mean difference in response between the two groups is only .06.

Moreover, the largest difference between any income and education group is only .23. Thus, the findings do not warrant inferences concerning the differential effect of income or education upon the behavioral expectations associated with the ill person.

TABLE 27. *Mean Response of Low-, Middle-, and High-Income Groups to Each Illness Condition in Each Behavioral Area*

Behavioral Area and Income Group	CRITICAL		WORSE		NOT UP TO PAR		BETTER		CONTROLLABLE		CHRONIC	
	In-come	Educa-tion	In-come	Educa-tion	In-come	Educa-tion	In-come	Educa-tion	In-come	Educa-tion	In-come	Educa-tion
A. Medical care												
Low	1.40	1.44	1.72	1.75	1.94	1.89	2.48	2.475	2.58	2.56	2.17	2.10
Middle	1.29	1.30	1.62	1.61	1.97	1.92	2.49	2.51	2.71	2.67	2.05	2.13
High	1.24	1.23	1.59	1.62	1.81	1.88	2.66	2.49	2.76	2.62	2.18	2.17
B. Physical Comfort												
Low	1.43	1.48	1.42	1.47	2.55	2.58	2.65	2.63	2.90	2.94	2.43	2.42
Middle	1.35	1.34	1.46	1.40	2.69	2.57	2.81	2.74	3.27	3.14	2.48	2.38
High	1.29	1.315	1.49	1.505	2.72	2.75	2.75	2.845	3.28	3.28	2.57	2.605
C. Social Responsibility												
Low	1.83	1.81	2.08	2.18	2.77	2.76	2.84	2.87	3.27	3.21	2.78	2.80
Middle	1.66	1.64	2.05	2.07	2.90	2.88	3.10	3.01	3.46	3.42	2.99	2.89
High	1.60	1.65	2.04	1.98	3.05	2.97	3.10	3.13	3.47	3.53	3.13	3.02
D. Information												
Low	1.62	1.63	1.81	1.85	2.45	2.41	2.41	2.55	2.59	2.53	2.51	2.53
Middle	1.45	1.48	1.55	1.62	2.45	2.49	2.50	2.46	2.63	2.72	2.55	2.49
High	1.26	1.28	1.61	1.54	2.49	2.36	2.79	2.56*	2.90	2.70	2.82	2.70

* This is the only difference approaching significance ($p < .05$).

The similarity between the income and educational analysis leads to the supposition that responses to the various illness states are determined primarily by a respondent's over-all socioeconomic status. If this is true a comparison of the low- and high-status groups should yield larger differences in response than did the educational and income comparisons. As anticipated, the differences between the low- and the high-status groups were consistently greater than the differences between either the income groups or the education groups.

For example, while there are no instances in which the differences between income and analogous educational groups are significantly greater than the differences between the high- and the low-status groups, in the following four instances the dif-

TABLE 28. *Mean Responses to the Behavioral Areas in Cluster 5 for Low and High Income, Education, and Income-Education Groups*

Behavioral Area and Group	CRITICAL			WORSE		
	In-come	Educa-tion	Income–Educa-tion	In-come	Educa-tion	Income–Educa-tion
A. Medical Care						
Low	1.40	1.44	1.51	1.72	1.75	1.81
High	1.24	1.23	1.25	1.59	1.62	1.61
Difference	.16	.21	.26	.13	.13	.20
B. Physical Comfort						
Low	1.43	1.47	1.53	1.42	1.47	1.52
High	1.29	1.315	1.28	1.49	1.505	1.515
Difference	.14	.155	.35	−.07	−.035	.005
C. Social Responsibility						
Low	1.83	1.81	2.02	2.08	2.18	2.215
High	1.60	1.65	1.66	2.04	1.98	2.15
Difference	.23	.16	.36	.04	.20	.065
D. Information						
Low	1.62	1.63	1.73	1.81	1.85	2.02
High	1.26	1.28	1.23	1.61	1.54	1.56
Difference	.36	.35	.50	.20	.31	.46
Mean Difference	*.22*	*.22*	*.37*	*.11*	*.17*	*.18*

ferences between the status groups are significantly greater ($p<.05$) than the differences between the income and educational groups: Illness Critical—Information; Illness Chronic—Information; Not Up to Par—Physical Comfort; Illness Controlled—Social Responsibility.

Furthermore, as shown in Table 30, in 17 out of the 24 instances in which differences were compared, the differences between the low-status and high-status groups are greater than either the differences between the income groups or the education groups. By chance it would be expected that the differences between the low-status and the high-status groups would be greater than the differences between both of the other groups in one-third of the comparisons. The fact that the socioeconomic status groups had greater differences in 70 per cent of the comparisons—an occur-

TABLE 29. *Mean Responses to the Behavioral Areas in Cluster 6 for Low and High Income, Education, and Income–Education Groups*

Behavioral Area and Group	NOT UP TO PAR			BETTER		
	In-come	Educa-tion	Income–Educa-tion	In-come	Educa-tion	Income–Educa-tion
A. Medical Care						
Low	1.94	1.89	1.89	2.48	2.475	2.395
High	1.81	1.88	1.89	2.66	2.49	2.605
Difference	.13	.01	.00	−.18	−.015	−.21
B. Physical Comfort						
Low	2.55	2.58	2.54	2.65	2.63	2.52
High	2.72	2.75	2.91	2.75	2.845	2.77
Difference	−.17	−.17	−.37	−.10	−.215	−.25
C. Social Responsibility						
Low	2.77	2.76	2.69	2.84	2.87	2.775
High	3.05	2.97	2.91	3.10	3.13	3.17
Difference	−.28	−.21	−.22	−.26	−.26	−.395
D. Information						
Low	2.45	2.41	2.42	2.41	2.55	2.54
High	2.49	2.36	2.40	2.79	2.56	2.77
Difference	−.04	.05	.02	−.38	−.01	−.23
Mean Difference	.15	.11	.15	.23	.125	.27

TABLE 29.—*Continued*

Behavioral Area and Group	CONTROLLABLE			CHRONIC		
	In-come	Educa-tion	Income–Educa-tion	In-come	Educa-tion	Income–Educa-tion
A. Medical Care						
Low	2.58	2.56	2.50	2.17	2.10	2.07
High	2.76	2.62	2.87	2.18	2.17	2.14
Difference	−.18	−.06	−.37	−.01	−.07	−.07
B. Physical Comfort						
Low	2.90	2.94	2.76	2.43	2.42	2.38
High	3.28	3.28	3.29	2.57	2.605	2.71
Difference	−.38	−.34	−.53	−.14	−.185	−.33
C. Social Responsibility						
Low	3.27	3.21	3.03	2.78	2.80	2.69
High	2.47	3.53	3.60	3.13	3.02	3.19
Difference	−.20	−.32	−.57	−.35	−.22	−.50
D. Information						
Low	2.51	2.53	2.45	2.50	2.53	2.45
High	2.90	2.70	2.90	2.82	2.70	3.01
Difference	−.39	−.17	−.45	−.32	−.17	−.56
Mean Difference	.29	.22	.48	.205	.16	.365

rence which would happen by chance less than once in one hundred times—lends further weight to my feeling that the responses to the illness conditions are determined to a greater extent by a person's general socioeconomic status than by either income or education.

Given the above findings it is not surprising to discover that the comparison of the high- and low-status groups further substantiates the responses to the existence of multimodal responses to illness conditions. As can be seen from Table 31, all differences in response to a given condition between these two socioeconomic status groups, with the exception of Condition *e* (Not up to par), are significant at $p<.01$. But, despite the finding that the tendency to treat the persons with the conditions in Cluster 6 as more dependent is somewhat greater for the low

TABLE 30. *Instances of Greatest Difference in Responses between Analogous Social and Economic Groups*

	Low Income and High Income	Grade School Education and College Education	Low Status and High Status	Total
Actual times with greatest difference	4	3.5*	17.5*	24
Expected times with greatest difference	8	8	8	24

* In one instance the Grade-school education and College education and Low Status and High Status groups tied for the greatest difference.

socioeconomic status group than for either the low-income or the grade school group, seriousness of the prognosis remains for all groups a major factor in determining the extent to which an ill person will be treated as a dependent. This conclusion is pointed up by the finding, shown in Table 31, that for the low-status group as well as the high-status group the tendency to treat the ill person as dependent increases as the prognosis becomes more uncertain and serious.

TABLE 31. *Mean Response by Socioeconomic Status Groups for Each Condition*

Condition	Low Status	High Status	Significance of Difference
Cluster 5 (Sick)			$p<$
c) Critical	1.70	1.355	.01
a) Worse	1.89	1.71	.01
Cluster 6 (Impaired)			
e) Not up to par	2.385	2.535	N.S.
b) Better	2.56	2.83	.01
f) Controlled	2.685	3.165	.01
d) Chronic	2.40	2.76	.01

In addition, the position, that the expectations Parsons associates with the sick role are determined more by the prognosis than by functional or physical incapacity, is supported by two facts: (1) there are no significant differences in the responses of either of the status groups to Condition *d* (Chronic) and Condition *e* (Not up to par), and (2) the tendency to treat the ill person as dependent is significantly greater in response to Condition *a* (Worse) and Condition *c* (Critical). This plus the finding that the greater tendency of the low-status group than of either the low-income or the grade school group to treat respondents with the conditions in Cluster 6 as more dependent does not mean that the group responds similarly to the conditions in Cluster 5 and Cluster 6. Further, the distinctions between conditions in Cluster 5 and 6 are not blurred even for the low-status group. In all instances there is a distinct and statistically significant tendency to treat conditions in Cluster 5 as more dependent than conditions in Cluster 6. This indicates fairly conclusively that while systematic socio-status differences in response occur, these differences are quantitative rather than qualitative.

The findings of the analysis, therefore, lead to the acceptance of:

Hypothesis 4: As the prognosis varies from controlled and known to unknown and serious, the tendency increases to exempt the ill person from social responsibility and from care of self, and to insure his obtaining technically competent help (i.e., the person will be treated as a dependent).

Hypothesis 5: Even in the presence of functional and physical impairment, the anticipated behavior toward the ill person will differ greatly depending upon whether the prognosis is non-serious and known, or serious and uncertain.

Hypothesis 6: As socioeconomic status decreases, the tendency increases to treat persons with illnesses that have a non-serious prognosis as dependent.

In addition to the acceptance of these hypotheses, the analysis revealed that all socioeconomic status groups associate two distinct sets of role expectations with illness. One set of role expectations, which adheres closely to those Parsons describes, becomes operative when the prognosis is uncertain and serious. The other set of role expectations, which tends to support independence, occurs when physical impairment is not accompanied by an uncertain or serious prognosis.

Behavioral Expectations Regarding the Role Relationships of the Sick Person

Given the findings in Chapter IV (that the tendency to define someone as sick is directly related to the uncertainty and seriousness of the prognosis) and the findings of this chapter (that the tendency to treat a person as dependent is directly related to the uncertainty and seriousness of the prognosis), it is apparent that, when someone occupies the status "sick," the over-all tendency is to treat him as a dependent. This finding throws light on general behavioral tendencies toward the sick person, but we must still determine the extent to which the tendencies are reflected in specific role relationships.

To investigate this problem, the respondents were asked the following questions:

Here are some statements people have made concerning a sick person. Which statement do you agree with most?

1. There is not much sense in following doctor's orders strictly because if you're supposed to get well, you will anyway.
2. A sick person can only do so much—it's really up to the doctor to get him well.
3. All a doctor can do is give the instructions; after that it's up to the patient.
4. A sick person knows better than a doctor what's really the matter with him, and it's up to him to decide whether to follow a doctor's orders or not.

Here's another list of statements about what a person can do when he is sick at home with something fairly serious. Which statement do you agree with most?

1. When a person is sick, he is helpless.

2. When a person is sick, there is very little he can do for himself.
3. When a person is sick, he can still do some things for himself.
4. When a person is sick, he can still do most things for himself.

Here's a final list. Again, a person is sick at home with something fairly serious. Tell me which statement describes what is most likely to happen?

1. When a person is sick, his family will leave him out of things.
2. When a person is sick, his family will keep family worries and problems from him.
3. When a person is sick, his family still counts on him to carry out some of his family duties and obligations.
4. When a person is sick, his family will make no important family decisions without his OK.

It should be noted that the role relationships referred to in these questions are the three dyadic role relationships which Parsons feels are particularly relevant to the sick role. In addition, each of the statements associated with a given role refers to one of the four possible reactions which Parsons implies occur when a person is sick. The first statement in each list refers to a feeling that one is helpless in the relationship—a tendency to view one's self as helpless and to reject the possibility of self-help. The second statement implies a dependent relationship—a tendency to give up some responsibility but with a residue of responsibility remaining. The third statement implies a tendency toward a normal relationship—a tendency to seek to maintain as far as possible the responsibilities inherent in the status "well." The final statement implies an overindependent role relationship—a tendency to demand more independence when sick than when well. Thus, as one moves from statement 1 to statement 4, the responses describe an increasingly independent role relationship.

When the responses to these questions are examined, it is found that two distinct response patterns emerge (see Table 32). The responses to the sick person–doctor dyad and the sick person–

TABLE 32. *Mean Response to Each Dyadic Role Relationship* (N=808)

Role Relationship	Mean Response
A. Sick person–Doctor	2.76
B. Sick person–Self	2.81
C. Sick person–Family	2.34

The difference between Sick person–Family role relationship and either of the other two dyadic role relationships is significant at $p<.01$.

self dyad tend to cluster around the third item, which implies independent or normal role relationships. On the other hand, it is found that responses to the sick person–family dyad cluster around the second item, which implies a dependent role relationship. Despite the fact that, in two of the three pairs of role relationships, there is a tendency toward independent role relationships, the findings do not contradict Parsons' statement that the sick person is treated as a dependent. Parsons points out that, while the sick person is relieved of daily activities, he has a social obligation to help himself and to cooperate as much as he can with the physician. Consequently, the finding that the sick person is expected to be somewhat independent in the sick person–doctor relationship and the sick person–self relationship, rather than contradicting Parsons, tends to support his theory.

Since two response patterns emerge for the three role pairs, the question remains: Do the responses represent a single statistical dimension? It was hypothesized that, when a person is defined as sick, there will be a high correlation between the appropriate patterns of dependence or independence in each of the dyadic relationships. To test this hypothesis, the responses to given role pairs were cluster analyzed. Not only did the items fail to cluster, but, as is shown in Table 33, the correlations among them are negligible.

The question then arises: Is the lack of correlation related to systematic socioeconomic variations in the response patterns to the three role pairs? To answer this question, the population was

TABLE 33. *Correlation Coefficients for*
Dyadic Role Relationships

Role Relationship	A	B	C
A. Sick person–Doctor	–	.07	.05
B. Sick person–Self		–	.15
C. Sick person–Family			–

divided into the income and education groups first used in Chapter IV. Table 34 shows that the only significant differences in the response patterns of the three income groups is the greater tendency of the high-income group to consider the sick person–self relationship as more independent than is the case for the middle- or the low-income groups.

The findings for the education analysis parallel the findings of the income analysis. Thus, we are unable to determine the differential effect of income, education, or a person's total socioeconomic status upon the response to the sick person–self role relationship. It can be stated, however, that the tendency to consider the sick person–self relationship as independent is directly related to factors associated with socioeconomic status. The fact that there is a systematic socioeconomic variation in response to the sick person–self relationship and not in the

TABLE 34. *Mean Response for Each Income Group*
*to Each Dyadic Role Relationship**

Role Relationship	Low Income (N=272)	Middle Income (N=327)	High Income (N=108)
A. Sick person–Doctor	2.77	2.84	2.84
B. Sick person–Self	2.63	2.89	3.00
C. Sick person–Family	2.43	2.43	2.46

* Differences between the low-income group and each of the two upper groups in response to the Sick person–Self dyad are the only significant differences between income groups ($p<.01$).

other relationships, and the fact that the central response tendency in the case of the sick person–family relationship differs from the central response tendency for the other two role relationships, explain, in part at least, why there is a lack of correlation between the response patterns for the three relationships.

The findings of this analysis of the behavioral expectations regarding the role relationships of the sick person lead, therefore, to the rejection of:

> *Hypothesis 7:* When a person is defined as sick, there will be a high correlation between the appropriate dependency or independency pattern in one dyadic relationship and the appropriate pattern in each of the other dyadic relationships.

There is little or no correlation between the appropriate dependency or independency pattern in one dyadic relationship and the appropriate dependency pattern in the other dyadic relationships.

The findings also lead to the rejection of:

> *Hypothesis 8:* As socioeconomic status decreases, the tendency increases to regard independence as the appropriate behavior of the sick person in each of the three dyadic role relationships.

Only in response to the sick person–self role relationship was there an inverse relationship between factors associated with socioeconomic status and the tendency to regard the appropriate behavior of the sick person as dependent.

Chapter Six

Conclusions

The concept of the sick role, developed by Talcott Parsons, has been widely referred to by medical sociologists and others, but until relatively recently it has primarily appeared in studies of an anthropological or psychological nature. One reason for the limited use of the concept is that it is based on an anthropological or unimodal conception of role. The effect of this unimodal conception has been to draw investigators' attention away from sociocultural variations in illness behavior. Furthermore, despite the fact that many researchers consider Parsons' concept of the sick role definitive, it has not been validated or effectively delineated. Until validation and delineation have been accomplished, the usefulness of the concept must be limited. In this study, therefore, the possibility that there are multimodal illness expectancies was explored and an attempt was made to delineate and distinguish the sick role from other types of behavior relevant to the ill person.

On the basis of an area probability sample of one thousand persons residing in New York City, the following hypotheses were tested:

Hypothesis	*Result*
1. There is an inverse relationship between socio-economic status and the importance of functional or physical incapacity as a factor in identifying someone as sick.	Accepted

2. In the absence of physical and functional inca-   Rejected
pacity, there is a direct relationship between socioeconomic status and the tendency to define someone
as sick on the basis of his being under a physician's
care.

3. The poorer or more uncertain the prognosis, the   Accepted
greater the tendency to define someone as sick.

4. As the prognosis varies from controlled and   Accepted
known to unknown and serious, the tendency increases to exempt the ill person from social responsibility and from care of self, and to insure his obtaining technically competent help (i.e., the person will
be treated as a dependent).

5. Even in the presence of functional and physical   Accepted
impairment, the anticipated behavior toward the ill
person will differ greatly depending upon whether
the prognosis is non-serious and known, or serious
and uncertain.

6. As socioeconomic status decreases, the tendency   Accepted
increases to treat persons with illnesses that have a
non-serious prognosis as dependent.

7. When a person is defined as sick, there will be a   Rejected
high correlation between the appropriate depend-
ency or independency pattern in one dyadic relationship and the appropriate pattern in each of the
other dyadic relationships.

8. As socioeconomic status decreases, the tendency   Rejected
increases to regard independence as the appropriate
behavior of the sick person in each of the three
dyadic role relationships.

On the basis of these and other findings presented in this study,
it was concluded that the criteria utilized to validate occupancy
of the statuses associated with these sets of role expectations
vary systematically between different socioeconomic groups. It

was found, for instance, that there is an inverse relationship between factors associated with socioeconomic status and the tendency to define someone as sick solely in terms of functional incapacity. However, the difference in the criteria used by various socioeconomic status groups to validate the status "sick" appears quantitative rather than qualitative. This conclusion is indicated by the fact that, for all socioeconomic groups, the major factor in defining someone as sick appears to be the prognosis.

The findings further revealed that, for each socioeconomic group, the factors which lead respondents to define someone as sick also lead respondents to treat the ill person as dependent or in Parsons' terms as "sick." In addition, when someone is defined as sick, all socioeconomic groups tend to respond to him in terms of similar behavioral expectations. This fact is indicated by the finding that there were no significant differences between socioeconomic groups in response to the questions concerning the sick person–doctor relationship or the sick person–family relationship. This lack of difference seems to imply that there is consensus throughout the population in terms of the behavioral expectations relevant to the sick role. Differences in role expectations regarding different illness states, therefore, appear to be related not to differing conceptions of the appropriate manner of treating the sick person, but rather to differing conceptions of who is and who is not sick.

One of the more important and unexpected findings of the study was that there are at least two distinct and unrelated statuses and complementary role expectations associated with illness states. One set of behavior expectancies, which was termed the "sick role," occurs when the prognosis is believed to be serious and uncertain. The other set of behavioral expectations was referred to as the "impaired role" and occurs when prognosis is believed to be known and non-serious. The initial set of role expectations adheres closely to Parsons' description of the sick role, while within the limitations of a given condition the second set of role expectations tends to support normal behavior. In sum, the role pressures relevant to the sick role serve to insulate and protect the ill person, while the role pressures relevant to the impaired role serve to aid and maintain normal activities and involvement. There is no inherent sequential relationship between the two roles, and it is possible to occupy either role without occupying the other.

Under conditions of more or less total helplessness, the ill person is of necessity defined as sick. But not only is extreme helplessness the exception rather than the rule in illness, many of the crucial illness decisions are made in the generally less helpless early and recuperative stages of an illness. Both because greater variations of response are possible and because of the importance of the decisions made in these stages, the distinctions between the "impaired" and the "sick" role appear most pertinent in the early and recuperative stages of an illness.

In concluding I think it's worthwhile to discuss briefly some of the implications of the findings. It is my belief that the appropriateness or inappropriateness of the role response to the ill person can delay, prevent or promote recovery—misappropriate responses can keep a person an invalid, delay seeking of care, or lead the ill person to attempt to function normally before he is able. Moreover, both the use of medical facilities and the effectiveness of treatment seem related to the role definitions employed. For instance, the findings show that when someone is defined as "impaired" not only is he denied certain supports but there is some discouragement of his seeking medical care. Inappropriateness of response is not solely due to individual miscalculations. The evidence indicates, for example, that lower-status persons have a tendency to treat persons with non-serious illnesses as more dependent than appears desirable by the standards of the middle- and upper-status groups.

As a general guide, the use of prognosis as the key to determining the social response to an illness condition seems eminently reasonable. But illness is a complicated phenomenon which, in the final analysis, must be treated on an individual basis. The person who appears most able to determine the appropriate role response is the physician. If illness is conceived of as a total process, then treatment must be conceived of as a total process and the patient's social environment must be considered a part of the treatment process. In addition to prescribing medical treatment the physician should prescribe the social response to the ill person. However, it is not enough for the doctor to prescribe a social response; just as he checks to see whether his medical prescriptions are being followed, he must determine, by judicious probing, if his social prescriptions are being followed. The prescribing of social response to an illness condition is something most doctors are reluctant to do because of lack of time and lack of knowledge. Nevertheless, social prescriptions are an essential part of the treatment process and cannot be delegated to those who have no role in that process. On the other hand, those of us interested in studying the social aspects of illness should attempt to provide physicians with the knowledge needed to make social prescriptions.

Particularly, there is a need for further information on the data cues that people employ as indicators of the anticipated consequences of an illness and on the effect of the acceptance or rejection of the "sick" or "impaired" role upon treatment. But while the above information will clarify many questions, the discrimination between the sick and the impaired role found in this investigation can provide initial guides for public health programs in general and physicians in particular in prescribing the social treatment of the ill person.

Appendix I

Research Procedures and
Methods of Analysis

Research Procedures and Methods of Analysis

A. *Sampling Procedure*

The city was represented by one hundred segments or interview areas for the probability sample. There were ten address listings for each segment, or one thousand addresses in all. Addresses in a given segment were concentrated in a single block or along each of two adjacent streets. Each interviewer was given a number of listing sheets convenient to the interviewer's home. To facilitate interviewing, all the listing sheets for one interviewer covered addresses within a small area. The procedure used in selecting the household to be interviewed follows:

Selection of Blocks

The selection of blocks was made with probability proportionate to the number of dwelling units in 1950 on the same block. In all cities which in 1950 had populations of 50,000 or more inhabitants, the Bureau of Census published data showing the number of dwelling units on each block in 1950. With these data it is possible to select blocks for inclusion in the sample in such a manner that every block within the city is given a probability of being selected proportionate to its size. Blocks that had no dwelling units in 1950 but could have had dwelling units at the time of the survey were taken care of by combining them with adjacent blocks prior to the selection. Thus, blocks that did not contain any dwellings in 1950 were also given a probability of being selected and also every dwelling unit within the four boroughs no matter if it was constructed after 1950 had a chance of being included in the sample.

Selection of Dwelling Units within Blocks

The final stage of selection of respondents was subsampling a previously prepared listing sheet of dwelling units in each block. The half-open interval technique was utilized. The interviewer was given a starting address and an ending address and was told to start interviewing with the first address, but not including the last address. This procedure up-dated listing sheets and made the design self-weighting.

An X-ing pattern for equal probabilities was utilized to select the respondent to be interviewed within each household.* The X-ing pattern on each enumeration sheet was covered with masking tape. The interviewer was told that, after enumerating the residents of a household, he was to remove the masking tape and arrange to interview the last person on the sheet whose name was followed by an X. The instructions for enumeration read as follows:

> Now obtain the following information about each occupant eighteen years of age or older and enter it in columns 3 through 5 of the table below. Before posting the name, find out whether this person is in the armed forces or has their real residence elsewhere. Exclude those persons for whom either of these situations applies from your listing. Also ask whether each young adult under 21 is going to school full-time (not working or otherwise independently occupied). Exclude such dependents. Enter or list information for men first from oldest to youngest and women afterwards from oldest to youngest.

As a check on the validity of the enumeration procedures, 25 per cent of each interviewer's enumerations were checked by a senior staff member. If an error occurred, the interview was invalidated, and the remainder of the interviewer's enumerations were checked. Before starting out, an interviewer knew where he was going to interview, but he did not know, until the persons living at a particular address had been enumerated, which particular person would be interviewed.

B. *Plan of Analysis and Statistical Procedures*

Hypothesis 1. There is an inverse relationship between socioeconomic status and the importance of functional or physical incapacity as a factor in identifying someone as sick.

Hypothesis 2. In the absence of physical and functional incapacity, there is a direct relationship between socioeconomic status and the tendency to define someone as sick on the basis of his being under a physician's care.

* To counterbalance the tendency for persons in small households to be overrepresented in the samples, questionnaire responses were weighted by household size.

Hypothesis 3. The poorer or more uncertain the prognosis, the greater the tendency to define someone as sick.

Relevant Questionnaire Items

Here's a list. Pick the word that best describes each condition I'm going to read to you.

handicapped, crippled, invalid, chronically ill, sick, all right, sickly

a) A person has a severe case of pneumonia? . . .
b) . . . had something a year ago and as a result lost the use of his legs?
c) . . . is recovering but not yet back to work?
d) . . . had something five years ago and since then cannot do strenuous work?
e) . . . has persistent pains in the stomach but can still work?
f) . . . has had arthritis for the past several years?
g) . . . is under a doctor's care but can work?
h) . . . has increasingly bad attacks of rheumatism?
i) . . . has an illness which keeps him in bed on and off? While it has not gotten worse, there appears little hope that it will improve?
j) . . . has been told that if he does not take it easy, he will have a severe attack?
k) . . . has had something which has left him deaf?
l) . . . is recovering but still in bed?

Main statistical technique used in testing Hypothesis 1, 2 and 3: z test.

In the examination of role patterns of the sick person (behavioral expectations of the sick role, dependency, and other patterns), the three aspects of role expectations which Parsons feels are important in the sick role were concentrated on: (1) expectations of exemptions from responsibility, (2) expectations of being physically taken care of, and (3) expectations regarding technically competent help.

Hypothesis 4. As the prognosis varies from controlled and known to unknown and serious, the tendency increases to exempt the ill person from social responsibility and from care of self, and to insure his obtaining technically competent help (i.e., the person will be treated as a dependent).

Hypothesis 5. Even in the presence of functional and physical impairment, the anticipated behavior toward the ill person will differ greatly depending upon whether the prognosis is non-serious and known, or serious and uncertain.

Hypothesis 6. As socioeconomic status decreases, the tendency increases to treat persons with illnesses that have a non-serious prognosis as dependent.

Relevant Questionnaire Items

I have here four lists containing some statements people have made about how to treat a sick person. I want you to read the list carefully, and tell me which statement describes the best thing to do when . . .

a) . . . a person's illness appears to be getting worse?

b) . . . a person appears to be getting better?

c) . . . the illness is critical?

d) . . . a person is suffering from a chronic illness (arthritis, rheumatism) or from the permanent effects of an illness (lameness)?

e) . . . a person complains over a period of time that they aren't feeling well (has aches or nausea or discomfort), can still work, but doesn't know why they aren't feeling up to par?

f) . . . a person has an illness, such as diabetes, and can go about his daily routine so long as he follows his doctor's orders and takes the right medicine?

List A.   Medical Care*

    1. See to it that he sees a doctor.

    2. Encourage him to see a doctor.

    3. Discourage him from running to a doctor with small aches and pains.

    4. See to it that he doesn't run to a doctor with small aches and pains.

List B.   Physical Comfort

    1. Give them a great deal of extra care.

    2. See to it that they are comfortable.

* The statements are listed in order of increasing independence (1 = maximum dependence, 4 = maximum independence). For the actual order of statements as presented to each respondent, see pp. 116-17. The actual order was determined by random selection.

3. Encourage them to do things for themselves.
4. Treat them like everybody else.

List C.   Social Responsibility
1. Make major decisions for them.
2. Keep responsibilities and worries from them.
3. Encourage them to do some sort of useful work.
4. Urge them to carry their daily responsibilities.

List D.   Information
1. Make sure that he tells you about any changes in his condition no matter how unimportant they seem.
2. Discourage him from bothering you about every little ache and pain.
3. Encourage him to tell you about any change in his condition no matter how unimportant they seem.
4. Steer him away from bothering you about every little ache and pain.

Main statistical technique used in testing:
Hypothesis 4: z test, correlation, and cluster analysis.
Hypothesis 5: z test and cluster analysis.
Hypothesis 6: z test.

Dyadic Role Relations. Parsons' three dyadic role relations (doctor–patient, family–patient, and self [ego]–patient) were analyzed in terms of the four reactions that he postulates occur when a person is sick.

1. Overindependence—tendency to demand more independence when sick than when well.
2. Normal independence—tendency to seek to maintain as far as possible the responsibilities inherent in the status "well".
3. Dependence—tendency to give up some responsibility but with a residue of responsibility remaining (Parson's sick role).
4. Self-pity—tendency to view one's self as helpless and to reject the possibility of self-help.

Hypothesis 7. When a person is defined as sick, there will be a high correlation between the appropriate dependency or independency pattern in one dyadic relationship and the appropriate pattern in each of the other dyadic relationships.

Hypothesis 8. As socioeconomic status decreases, the tendency increases to regard independence as the appropriate behavior of the sick person in each of the three dyadic role relationships.

Relevant Questionnaire Items

Here are some statements people have made concerning a sick person. Which statement do you agree with most?*

1. There is not much sense in following a doctor's orders strictly because if you're supposed to get well, you will anyway.
2. A sick person can only do so much—it's really up to the doctor to get him well.
3. All a doctor can do is give the instructions, after that it's up to the patient.
4. A sick person knows better than a doctor what's really the matter with him, and it's up to him to decide whether to follow a doctor's orders or not.

Here's another list of statements about what a person can do when he is sick at home with something fairly serious. Which statement do you agree with most?

1. When a person is sick, he is helpless.
2. When a person is sick, there is very little he can do for himself.
3. When a person is sick, he can still do some things for himself.
4. When a person is sick, he can still do most things for himself.

Here's a final list. Again a person is sick at home with something fairly serious. Tell me which statement describes what is most likely to happen?

1. When a person is sick, his family will leave him out of things.
2. When a person is sick, his family will keep family worries and problems from him.
3. When a person is sick, his family still counts on him to carry out some of his family duties and obligations.
4. When a person is sick, his family will make no important family decisions without his OK.

---

* The statements are listed in order of increasing independence (1 = helpless or self-pity, 2 = dependence, 3 = normal independence, 4 = overindependence). For the actual order of statements see pp. 119-20. The order was determined by random selection.

Main statistical technique used in testing:

Hypothesis 7: cluster analysis.

Hypothesis 8: z test.

Throughout the analysis an attempt was made to examine four factors: differences in response between groups, differences in consensus, the extent to which responses represent a uni-dimensional attitude or response, and the degree of relationship between responses. The z test was used to determine whether differences in responses between groups were significant. This technique assumes that the distributions tested come from the same population.

$$z = \frac{X_1 - X_2}{\dfrac{S_1^2 - S_2^2}{N_1 - N_2}}$$

To test consensus or variance in response, the F test was employed.

$$F = \frac{S_1^2}{S_2^2}$$

The principal limitation of this technique is that variables with different ranges cannot be compared. This limitation, however, did not prove a drawback in this study because we were study-ing consensus regarding the same variable or variables with similar response possibilities.

The product–moment correlation was used to examine the degree of relationship between variables.

$$r = \frac{\Sigma\, xy - \overline{xy}}{N\ \sigma_x\ \sigma_y}$$

The only major limitation in use of this technique is that ranges should be equal. While this limitation on the use of the product–moment correlation did not prove a drawback in the analysis of consensus, it posed a more difficult problem. Since the variables used differed in possible range, the interpretation of results required considerable care. The general tendency is for correlations between variables of different ranges to be lower than thcy would normally be if the ranges were similar. For convenience in interpreting the meanings of the correlations, the variables were divided into three groups: wide range, medium range, and short range.

Wide-range variables
Illness getting worse
Illness getting better
Illness critical
Illness chronic
Person not up to par
Illness controlled
Seeking medical care
Home care
Work and responsibility
Information

Medium-range variables
Education of respondent
Income of main wage-earner

Short-range variables
Dependency in doctor–patient relationship
Dependency in family–patient relationship
Dependency in patient–self relationship

To summarize, correlations among variables of the same range group are more valid measures of closeness and can be taken more literally than correlations of wide-range variables with variables of shorter ranges. This last type of correlation is deflated because of the range difference. Thus, while the relationship between variables of different ranges can be demonstrated, the degree of relationship cannot be specified.

Cluster analysis was used to examine the extent to which responses represented a unidimensional attitude. This technique is really an extension of correlation. Once correlations have been obtained, we have some idea of the relationship between two variables. But if we seek to examine relationships among the many variables in order to uncover patterns inherent in the data, an extension technique, such as cluster analysis, is needed.

The purpose of cluster analysis is to group correlations of variables into "clusters" or basic statistical dimensions. From these, it is possible to derive indices of grouped variables that represent combinations of similar variables in clustered arrangement. The technique of cluster analysis groups items into dimensions, starting with the highest correlation of a series and proceeding with correlations in order of their magnitude, and computes the ratio of the mean of correlations within a cluster to the mean of the correlations remaining. This ratio, called the "B-coefficient," serves as a measure for the degree of the variable's "belonging" in a particular cluster.

Cluster analysis has certain limitations. A variable can appear in only one cluster and thus the significance of relationship in another cluster cannot be ascertained. However, if the B-coefficient is high, the variable is shown to have the "greatest" similarity to the other variables in this cluster. The second limitation is that the criteria for starting and stopping clusters are fairly arbitrary. The highest correlation in a series might be produced by specious factors. Further, there are no rigorous mathematical limits to determine the stopping of clusters. Rather a fairly substantial decrease, on the order of .20, is accepted as an indication that new variables are not contributing to clustering strength.

C. *Excerpts from Interview Manual*

1. *Presenting the Study*

There are certain things you should tell all respondents and there are certain general approaches that we feel are preferable to others. . . . Most important in this regard is your general identification of the nature of the study. Identify it as a study of how people feel about medical matters and about their own experiences with medical matters.

Avoid going into elaborate discussion of substantive aspects of the questionnaire in this preliminary talk. Don't present yourself, or the study, as advocates of a great deal of medical care, or modern medicine, or anything in particular, but simply as a group that feels the need for knowledge about how people feel on these matters. Present yourself, and the study, as neutral on all debatable health questions, and above all discourage any suspicion that we are trying to "check up" on people's health practices according to some preconceived schedule of "good" health practices.

2. *About Interviewing*

All interviews are to be conducted face to face with each respondent. *Never* interview anyone over the phone.

The respondent should never be permitted to read the questionnaire, or to fill it out himself. The interviewer asks the questions and records the person's answers. Never interview people in groups.

Try to avoid interviewing any person in the presence of another. *No substitutes or assistants* are allowed to do your work. If you cannot do the assignment yourself, contact the field supervisor immediately and hold all materials until you hear from him.

3. *How to Interview*

Your attitude at all times should be friendly, conversational, and impartial. Take all opinions in stride. *Never* show surprise at a person's answer, nor reveal your own opinions.

Do *not* explain a question or elaborate upon it unless so instructed. If the respondent does not understand the question, repeat it slowly with proper emphasis. Your survey specifications suggest specific explanatory probes.

Do not accept as final answers replies that do not specifically answer the question. In such cases, repeat the question, or tell the respondent you're not quite sure what he means.

Avoid qualified answers ("Well, it depends") by pressing for an opinion ("Well, taking everything into consideration," or "On the basis of the way things look now").

Never suggest a possible answer, nor help the respondent to arrive at any particular answer. Let him express his own opinions in his own way.

4. *Rules for Good Interviewing*

The main task in interviewing is to take every precaution to make sure that you get a clear, complete, and unambiguous statement of your respondent's ideas. Before you can confidently circle a pre-coded response, you must ask yourself whether the respondent has given a complete answer. Don't accept vague and unclear answers here or in the open-ended questions. Before you can leave an open-ended question and go on to the next topic, you must ask yourself the same questions.

Probing is important for both the pre-coded and the open-ended question. While you do not have to record the verbatim answer, you are still responsible for all the probing (continued neutral questioning) needed to get a satisfactory answer to pre-coded questions. You'll find, of course, that most pre-coded questions need less intensive probing than do the open-ended questions, but they will often need probing.

Most interviewers find the open-ended question somewhat more difficult and therefore more challenging than the pre-coded question. On every one of the open-ended questions, the general goal is to *find out exactly what the respondent is thinking,* both in relation to the general objectives of the survey and the specific purposes of that question. Your objective is to draw the person out, and to get him to express all of his ideas before leaving that question and going on to the next one. It is not enough simply to get an answer from the respondent. Instead, you must follow up what the respondent says, using probes to get him to expand and clarify his answer, until you are sure that you have the entire picture of the way the respondent thinks about the question.

Never suggest answers to your respondents. ALWAYS use probes like:

How do you mean?
Can you give me an example?
What do you have in mind?
Why do you say that?
Could you explain a little?
Do you have any other things in mind?

Or you can repeat the respondent's own words with a rising inflection, to suggest that you are not sure of exactly what he means. DON'T SUGGEST ANSWERS. The new interviewer may find it hard not to suggest answers, for in normal conversation we often do so without realizing it. While one may think of interviewing as a friendly conversation, it is a rather artificial one. In most conversations it's quite common for a person who is not certain what his partner means by an expression to suggest the meaning.

D. *Order and Method of Presentation of Questionnaire Items*

Q. 68. I have here four lists containing some statements people have made about how to treat a sick person. (HAND "LIST A" TO RESPONDENT. READ QUESTION, USING EACH OF THE SIX COMPLETIONS BELOW IN TURN. CIRCLE RESPONDENT'S CHOICES FOR "BEST THING TO DO," FROM LIST A, IN TABLE ON RIGHT-HAND PAGE.)

A. I want you to read the list carefully, and tell me which statement describes the best thing to do when . . .

    (a) . . . a person's illness appears to be getting worse?

    (b) . . . a person appears to be getting better?

    (c) . . . the illness is critical?

    (d) . . . a person is suffering from a chronic illness (arthritis, rheumatism) or from the permanent effects of an illness (lameness)?

    (e) . . . a person complains over a period of time that he isn't feeling well (has aches or nausea or discomfort), can still work, but doesn't know why he isn't feeling up to par?

    (f) . . . a person has an illness, such as diabetes, and can go about his daily routine so long as he follows his doctor's orders and takes the right medicine?

B. (FOLLOW IDENTICAL PROCEDURE FOR "B" AS FOR "A," EXCEPT SUBSTITUTE "LIST B" FOR "LIST A.")

C. (AS FOR "A" and "B," SUBSTITUTE "LIST C.")

D. (AS FOR "A," "B" and "C," SUBSTITUTING "LIST D.")

THE BEST THING

LIST A	(a)	(b)	(c)	(d)	(e)	(f)
a) Encourage him to see a doctor	2	2	2	2	2	2
b) Discourage him from running to a doctor with small aches and pains	3	3	3	3	3	3
c) See to it that he sees a doctor	1	1	1	1	1	1
d) See to it that he doesn't run to a doctor with small aches and pains	4	4	4	4	4	4
D.K.	0	0	0	0	0	0
N.A.	x	x	x	x	x	x

LIST B	(a)	(b)	(c)	(d)	(e)	(f)
a) Give them a great deal of extra care	1	1	1	1	1	1
b) Encourage them to do things for themselves	3	3	3	3	3	3
c) See to it that they are comfortable	2	2	2	2	2	2
d) Treat them like everybody else	4	4	4	4	4	4
D.K.	0	0	0	0	0	0
N.A.	x	x	x	x	x	x

LIST C	(a)	(b)	(c)	(d)	(e)	(f)
a) Encourage them to do some sort of useful work	3	3	3	3	3	3
b) Keep responsibilities and worries from them	2	2	2	2	2	2
c) Make major decisions for them	1	1	1	1	1	1
d) Urge them to carry their daily responsibilities	4	4	4	4	4	4
D.K.	0	0	0	0	0	0
N.A.	x	x	x	x	x	x

LIST D	(a)	(b)	(c)	(d)	(e)	(f)
a) Steer him away from bothering you about every little ache and pain	4	4	4	4	4	4
b) Make sure that he tells you about any changes in his condition no matter how unimportant they may seem	1	1	1	1	1	1
c) Discourage him from bothering you about every little ache and pain	3	3	3	3	3	3
d) Encourage him to tell you about any changes in his condition no matter how unimportant they seem	2	2	2	2	2	2
D.K.	0	0	0	0	0	0
N.A.	x	x	x	x	x	x

Q. 69. A. Here's a list. Pick the word that best describes each condition I'm going to read to you. A person . . . (HAND CARD TO RESPONDENT. CIRCLE THE APPROPRIATE CODE FOR EACH "WORD CHOICE," "A" FOR CONDITION "a/" TO "1/")

WORD CHOICES

1) handicapped	3) invalid	5) sick	7) sickly
2) crippled	4) chronically ill	6) all right	

B. (AFTER YOU HAVE ASKED "A" FOR ALL CONDITIONS, ASK "B" FOR EACH CONDITION WHERE "SICK," CODE 5 IN "A," HAS NOT BEEN PICKED.) Would you say the following are sick or not sick?

a) . . . has a severe case of pneumonia?

A. (WORD CHOICES)	hand.	crip.	inv.	chron.	sick	all r.	sickly	DK
	1	2	3	4	5	6	7	8

B. (SICKNESS)	sick	not sick	DK	"5" circled already in "A"
	0	1	2	x

b) . . . had something a year ago and as a result lost the use of his legs?

A. (WORD CHOICES)	hand.	crip.	inv.	chron.	sick	all r.	sickly	DK
	1	2	3	4	5	6	7	8

B. (SICKNESS)	sick	not sick	DK	"5" circled already in "A"
	0	1	2	x

c) . . . is recovering but not yet back to work?

A. (WORD CHOICES)	hand.	crip.	inv.	chron.	sick	all r.	sickly	DK
	1	2	3	4	5	6	7	8

B. (SICKNESS)	sick	not sick	DK	"5" circled already in "A"
	0	1	2	x

d) . . . had something five years ago and since then cannot do strenuous work?

A. (WORD CHOICES)	hand.	crip.	inv.	chron.	sick	all r.	sickly	DK
	1	2	3	4	5	6	7	8

B. (SICKNESS)	sick	not sick	DK	"5" circled already in "A"
	0	1	2	x

e) . . . has persistent pains in the stomach but can still work?

A. (WORD CHOICES)	hand.	crip.	inv.	chron.	sick	all r.	sickly	DK
	1	2	3	4	5	6	7	8

B. (SICKNESS)	sick	not sick	DK	"5" circled already in "A"
	0	1	2	x

f) . . . has had arthritis for the past several years?

A. (WORD CHOICES)	hand.	crip.	inv.	chron.	sick	all r.	sickly	DK
	1	2	3	4	5	6	7	8

B. (SICKNESS)	sick	not sick	DK	"5" circled already in "A"
	0	1	2	x

g) . . . is under a doctor's care but can work?

A. (WORD CHOICES)	hand.	crip.	inv.	chron.	sick	all r.	sickly	DK
	1	2	3	4	5	6	7	8

B. (SICKNESS)	sick	not sick	DK	"5" circled already in "A"
	0	1	2	x

h) . . . has increasingly bad attacks of rheumatism?

| A. (WORD CHOICES) | hand. 1 | crip. 2 | inv. 3 | chron. 4 | sick 5 | all r. 6 | sickly 7 | DK 8 |

| B. (SICKNESS) | sick 0 | not sick 1 | DK 2 | "5" circled already in "A" x |

i) . . . has an illness which keeps him in bed on and off. While it has not gotten worse, there appears little hope that it will improve?

| A. (WORD CHOICES) | hand. 1 | crip. 2 | inv. 3 | chron. 4 | sick 5 | all r. 6 | sickly 7 | DK 8 |

| B. (SICKNESS) | sick 0 | not sick 1 | DK 2 | "5" circled already in "A" x |

j) . . . has been told that if he does not take it easy, he will have a severe attack?

| A. (WORD CHOICES) | hand. 1 | crip. 2 | inv. 3 | chron. 4 | sick 5 | all r. 6 | sickly 7 | DK 8 |

| B. (SICKNESS) | sick 0 | not sick 1 | DK 2 | "5" circled already in "A" x |

k) . . . has had something which has left him deaf?

| A. (WORD CHOICES) | hand. 1 | crip. 2 | inv. 3 | chron. 4 | sick 5 | all r. 6 | sickly 7 | DK 8 |

| B. (SICKNESS) | sick 0 | not sick 1 | DK 2 | "5" circled already in "A" x |

l) . . . is recovering but still in bed?

| A. (WORD CHOICES) | hand. 1 | crip. 2 | inv. 3 | chron. 4 | sick 5 | all r. 6 | sickly 7 | DK 8 |

| B. (SICKNESS) | sick 0 | not sick 1 | DK 2 | "5" circled already in "A" x |

Q. 83. Here are some statements people have made concerning a sick person. Which statement do you agree with most?

(HAND CARD TO RESPONDENT) List I

AGREE MOST

1) All a doctor can do is give the instructions, after that it's up to the patient. 3

2) There is not much sense in following doctor's orders strictly because if you're supposed to get well, you will anyway. 1

3) A sick person knows better than a doctor what's really the matter with him, and it's up to him to decide whether to follow a doctor's orders or not   4

4) A sick person can only do so much—it's really up to the doctor to get him well.   2

                         DK   0

                         NA   x

Here's another list of statements about what a person can do when he is sick at home with something fairly serious. Which statement do you agree with most?

	AGREE MOST
(HAND CARD TO RESPONDENT) List II	
1) When a person is sick, he can still do most things for himself.	4
2) When a person is sick, there is very little he can do for himself.	2
3) When a person is sick, he can still do some things for himself.	3
4) When a person is sick, he is helpless.	1
DK	0
NA	x

Here's a final list. Again, a person is sick at home with something fairly serious. Tell me which statement describes what is most likely to happen?

	AGREE MOST
(HAND CARD TO RESPONDENT.) List III	
1) When a person is sick, his family will make no important family decisions without his OK.	4
2) When a person is sick, his family will keep family worries and problems from him.	2
3) When a person is sick, his family will leave him out of things.	1
4) When a person is sick, his family still counts on him to carry out some of his family duties and obligations.	3
DK	0
NA	x

Factual Data

Q. 6. A. What was the name of the last school you attended? (SPECIFY)

B. What was the last grade (or year) you completed in that school?

Grammar School	0–4 years	0
	5–6 years	1
	7–8 years	2
High School	9–11 years	3
	12 years	4
College	1–3 years	5
	4 or more years	6
	DK	7
	NA	8

C. (HIGH SCHOOL ONLY) Was this an academic, vocational, or commercial high school? (IF SCHOOL WAS MIXED, ASK WHAT COURSE RESPONDENT TOOK AND CODE ACCORDINGLY.)

Academic	0
Vocational	1
Commercial	2
DK	3
NA	4
	x

Q. 9. How much income does the main wage-earner earn?

Under $1,000	0
$1,000–$1,999	1
$2,000–$2,999	2
$3,000–$3,999	3
$4,000–$4,999	4
$5,000–$7,499	5
$7,500–$9,999	6
$10,000–$14,999	7
$15,000–$19,999	8
$20,000 and plus	9
DK	X
NA	Y

Appendix II

Source Tables for Chapter IV

Source Tables for Chapter IV

TABLE 1

Per Cent of Persons (N=61) with Income $7,500 and Over and More than 12 Years Education Who Define a Given Description as Sick or Not Sick

Description	Sick	Not Sick	No Answer or Don't Know
A. Has pneumonia	100	....	....
I. Illness keeps him in bed on and off	96	4	....
H. Increasingly bad rheumatism	86	13	1
E. Persistent pains in stomach, can work	72	25	3
L. Recovering but in bed	69	25	5
F. Has arthritis	55	38.5	6
C. Recovering but not yet back to work	57	41.5	1.5
J. Must take it easy	51	49	....
G. Under doctor's care, can work	41	54	5
D. Had something five years ago and since then cannot do strenuous work	32	65	3
B. Lost use of legs	16	82	1.5
K. Is deaf	8.5	91.5	....

TABLE 2

Per Cent of Persons (N=122) with Income Under $4,000 and with 0–8 Years Education Who Define a Given Description as Sick or Not Sick

Description	Sick	Not Sick	No Answer or Don't Know
A. Has pneumonia	93	4	3.5
I. Illness keeps him in bed on and off	87	6	7
H. Increasingly bad rheumatism	81.5	11	7
F. Has arthritis	79	14	7
J. Must take it easy	78	15	7
K. Persistent pains in stomach, can work	76	17	7
L. Recovering but in bed	70	23	7
D. Had something five years ago and since then cannot do strenuous work	64.5	26	10
G. Under doctor's care, can work	63	28	9
C. Recovering but not yet back to work	63	30	7
B. Lost use of legs	48	45	7
K. Is deaf	45	48	7

TABLE 3

*Per Cent of Persons (N=272) with Income Under $4,000 Who Define
a Given Description as Sick or Not Sick*

Description	Sick	Not Sick	No Answer or Don't Know
A. Has pneumonia	95	2	2.5
I. Illness keeps him in bed on and off	90	6	5
H. Increasingly bad rheumatism	82.5	12	5
E. Persistent pains in stomach, can work	77	18	5
J. Must take it easy	76	19	5
L. Recovering but in bed	73	22	5
F. Has arthritis	73	21	5
C. Recovering but not yet back to work	66	30	4
G. Under doctor's care, can work	64	30	6
D. Had something five years ago and since then cannot do strenuous work	57	36	7
B. Lost use of legs	40	54	6
K. Is deaf	34	62	3

TABLE 4

*Per Cent of Persons (N=327) with $4,000–$7,499 Income Who
Define a Given Description as Sick or Not Sick*

Description	Sick	Not Sick	No Answer or Don't Know
A. Has pneumonia	99	....	1
I. Illness keeps him in bed on and off	94	3	3
H. Increasingly bad rheumatism	85	12	3
E. Persistent pains in stomach, can work	79	19	2
J. Must take it easy	79	17	4
L. Recovering but in bed	75	22.5	2
F. Has arthritis	69.5	27	4
C. Recovering but not yet back to work	68	30.5	2
G. Under doctor's care, can work	55	40	5
D. Had something five years ago and since then cannot do strenuous work	53	45	2
B. Lost use of legs	26	73	1
K. Is deaf	18	81	1

TABLE 5

Per Cent of Persons (N=108) with Income $7,500 and Over Who Define a Given Description as Sick or Not Sick

Description	Sick	Not Sick	No Answer or Don't Know
A. Has pneumonia	100	....	....
I. Illness keeps him in bed on and off	94	5	1
H. Increasingly bad rheumatism	82	16	2
E. Persistent pains in stomach, can work	79.5	18	3
L. Recovering but in bed	67	30	3
J. Must take it easy	59.5	40	1
F. Has arthritis	59	36	5
C. Recovering but not yet back to work	57	41	2
G. Under doctor's care, can work	42	53	4
D. Had something five years ago and since then cannot do strenuous work	38	61	2
B. Lost use of legs	20.5	79	1
K. Is deaf	7	92	1

TABLE 6

Per Cent of Persons (N=240) with 0–8 Years Education Who Define a Given Description as Sick or Not Sick

Description	Sick	Not Sick	No Answer or Don't Know
A. Has pneumonia	95	2	3
I. Illness keeps him in bed on and off	89	5	5.5
H. Increasingly bad rheumatism	82	12	6
E. Persistent pains in stomach, can work	77	18	5
J. Must take it easy	77	18	5
L. Recovering but in bed	77	19	4
F. Has arthritis	76	19	5
C. Recovering but not yet back to work	67	26.5	6
G. Under doctor's care, can work	63	30	6.5
D. Had something five years ago and since then cannot do strenuous work	63	30	6
B. Lost use of legs	45	51	5
K. Is deaf	39	57	4

TABLE 7

Per Cent of Persons (N=392) with 9–12 Years Education Who Define a Given Description as Sick or Not Sick

Description	Sick	Not Sick	No Answer or Don't Know
A. Has pneumonia	98.5	0.5	1
I. Illness keeps him in bed on and off	93	4	....
H. Increasingly bad rheumatism	84	13	3
E. Persistent pains in stomach, can work	79.5	18	2
J. Must take it easy	78	18.5	3
F. Has arthritis	70	26	4
L. Recovering but in bed	69	28	3
C. Recovering but not yet back to work	63	35	2
D. Had something five years ago and since then cannot do strenuous work	54	44	2.5
G. Under doctor's care, can work	52	43	4.5
B. Lost use of legs	29	67	4
K. Is deaf	19	80	1

TABLE 8

Per Cent of Persons (N=163) with More than 12 Years Education Who Define a Given Description as Sick or Not Sick

Description	Sick	Not Sick	No Answer or Don't Know
A. Has pneumonia	100	....	....
I. Illness keeps him in bed on and off	93	3	4
H. Increasingly bad rheumatism	87	12.5	1
E. Persistent pains in stomach, can work	79	18	3
L. Recovering but in bed	78	18	4
C. Recovering but not yet back to work	66	32.5	1.5
F. Has arthritis	62	34	3
J. Must take it easy	59	36	5
G. Under doctor's care, can work	52	43	5
D. Had something five years ago and since then cannot do strenuous work	37	60	3
B. Lost use of legs	15	82	3
K. Is deaf	11	86	2

Appendix III

Source Tables for Chapter V

Source Tables for Chapter V

TABLE 1

Percentage Distribution of Total Responses (N=808) by Illness Condition Regarding Medical Care

Response	Critical	Worse	Not Up to Par	Recovering	Controlled	Chronic
Don't know	0.8	0.7	1.6	5.3	9.0	2.5
See to it that he sees a doctor	72.6	37.9	24.1	14.4	12.7	27.0
Encourage him to see a doctor	21.7	58.2	63.9	32.1	26.4	42.4
Discourage him from running to a doctor with small aches and pains	1.0	.9	3.7	31.3	31.0	16.0
See to it that he doesn't run to a doctor with small aches and pains	1.5	.8	4.4	14.4	17.9	10.6
No answer	2.4	1.6	2.2	2.5	3.0	1.8

TABLE 2

Percentage Distribution of Total Responses (N=808) by Illness Condition Regarding Physical Comfort

Response	Critical	Worse	Not Up to Par	Recov- ering	Con- trolled	Chronic
Don't know	1.5	1.7	8.3	1.4	2.6	1.8
Give them a great deal of extra care	69.7	66.8	18.4	6.9	11.0	17.7
See to it that they are comfortable	22.6	23.0	22.4	22.8	9.7	35.8
Encourage them to do things for themselves	1.2	3.4	19.6	55.2	27.6	24.1
Treat them like everybody else	1.7	2.7	26.2	11.1	45.7	17.2
No answer	3.3	2.4	5.0	2.6	3.4	3.3

TABLE 3

Percentage Distribution of Total Responses (N=808) by Illness Condition Regarding Social Responsibility

Response	Critical	Worse	Not Up to Par	Recovering	Controlled	Chronic
Don't know	2.4	2.9	9.1	1.6	4.4	4.1
Make major decisions for them	40.2	11.0	6.4	3.9	2.8	6.5
Keep responsibilities and worries from them	48.3	70.7	24.6	14.2	7.8	20.9
Encourage them to do some sort of useful work	3.4	8.6	24.3	52.1	26.3	39.1
Urge them to carry their daily responsibilities	2.0	3.4	30.6	24.5	55.0	26.2
No answer	3.6	3.4	5.0	3.6	3.7	3.2

TABLE 4

Percentage Distribution of Total Responses (N=808) by Illness Condition Regarding Information

Response	Critical	Worse	Not Up to Par	Recovering	Controlled	Chronic
Don't know	3.5	2.6	7.1	3.2	5.3	3.9
Make sure that he tells you about any changes in his condition	61.2	47.7	19.5	21.4	16.9	19.3
Encourage him to tell you about any changes in his condition	26.5	38.9	29.7	25.4	22.1	25.5
Discourage him from bothering you about every little ache and pain	2.3	1.7	20.5	24.0	25.8	24.1
Steer him away from bothering you about every ache and pain	2.1	4.9	18.4	22.2	25.1	22.8
No answer	4.4	4.9	4.9	3.9	4.9	4.4

TABLE 5

Per Cent of Responses by Illness Condition Regarding Medical Care for Education Groups

Response and Education Group*	Critical	Worse	Not Up to Par	Better	Con-trolled	Chronic
Don't know						
Grade School	-2.0	2.0	4.3	2.9	6.9	4.3
High School	(.2)	(.2)	(.6)	(5.2)	(8.7)	(1.8)
College	.3	—	—	9.2	13.9	1.7
See to it that he sees a doctor						
Grade School	63.9	30.4	27.0	17.4	15.9	27.2
High School	(74.3)	(40.3)	(23.6)	(14.0)	(11.9)	(28.5)
College	81.8	42.2	21.1	10.7	9.8	42.2
Encourage him to see a doctor						
Grade School	27.0	62.1	56.8	30.4	30.3	42.1
High School	(21.2)	(57.6)	(64.7)	(32.5)	(23.7)	(40.1)
College	15.3	55.2	72.5	33.8	25.7	48.3
Discourage him from running to a doctor with small aches and pains						
Grade School	1.4	1.6	3.1	27.0	24.9	11.8
High School	(1.0)	(.6)	(4.3)	(32.1)	(33.7)	(17.0)
College	.6	.6	3.5	36.7	33.8	20.2
See to it that he doesn't run to a doctor with small aches and pains						
Grade School	1.8	.6	4.3	17.2	16.9	10.6
High School	(1.1)	(.4)	(5.3)	(14.7)	(20.1)	(11.7)
College	2.0	2.0	2.6	9.2	15.3	8.7
No answer						
Grade School	3.9	3.3	4.3	4.9	5.5	3.9
High School	(2.2)	(.8)	(1.4)	(1.4)	(1.8)	(.8)
College	—	—	.3	.3	1.4	—

* N = 240 for Grade School Group, 392 for High School Group, and 163 for College Group.

TABLE 6

Per Cent of Responses by Illness Condition Regarding Physical Comfort for Education Groups

Response and Education Group*	Critical	Worse	Not Up to Par	Better	Controlled	Chronic
Don't know						
Grade School	3.1	2.9	11.0	2.9	4.3	3.7
High School	—	(.7)	(6.1)	(.6)	(2.0)	(.7)
College	1.4	2.3	9.2	1.2	1.4	1.7
Give them a great deal of extra care						
Grade School	64.9	62.5	19.6	11.2	12.7	17.8
High School	(71.5)	(71.2)	(19.3)	(6.0)	(11.0)	(20.5)
College	72.5	61.8	11.8	1.7	6.1	8.7
See to it that they are comfortable						
Grade School	20.2	24.9	16.3	20.8	8.4	33.7
High School	(24.3)	(20.9)	(24.4)	(23.0)	(11.0)	(36.3)
College	23.1	26.3	28.3	25.4	6.1	40.5
Encourage them to do things for themselves						
Grade School	2.2	2.7	21.4	47.0	31.0	20.0
High School	(.4)	(2.3)	(20.9)	(59.8)	(26.2)	(25.1)
College	1.2	7.2	14.7	56.9	27.5	28.9
Treat them like everybody else						
Grade School	1.8	1.4	23.1	11.4	34.9	17.1
High School	(2.2)	(3.9)	(25.5)	(1.0)	(48.9)	(16.2)
College	.6	2.0	33.5	14.2	55.2	19.4
No answer						
Grade School	7.1	5.5	8.6	6.7	8.6	7.6
High School	(1.6)	(1.0)	(3.6)	(.5)	(.8)	(1.1)
College	1.2	.3	2.3	.6	1.2	.9

* N = 240 for Grade School Group, 392 for High School Group, and 163 for College Group.

TABLE 7

Per Cent of Responses by Illness Condition Regarding Social Responsibility for Education Groups

Response and Education Groups*	Critical	Worse	Not Up to Par	Better	Controlled	Chronic
Don't know						
Grade School	4.9	4.3	10.2	3.5	7.4	8.4
High School	(1.0)	(2.3)	(8.1)	(.7)	(3.3)	(2.0)
College	2.3	2.3	9.8	1.2	2.9	3.2
Make major decisions for them						
Grade School	37.4	9.0	9.2	5.9	3.9	8.6
High School	(43.3)	(11.1)	(5.5)	(4.1)	(2.9)	(5.7)
College	38.4	14.2	4.0	.9	1.2	4.9
Keep responsibilities and worries from them						
Grade School	40.2	62.1	22.9	17.4	9.2	19.4
High School	(50.3)	(76.6)	(26.4)	(13.4)	(7.9)	(24.4)
College	54.3	70.2	24.0	11.8	5.8	14.7
Encourage them to do some sort of useful work						
Grade School	7.3	13.5	21.9	42.3	25.5	31.8
High School	(2.0)	(5.8)	(25.5)	(57.3)	(26.8)	(40.6)
College	1.4	7.5	24.0	55.5	24.0	46.5
Urge them to carry their daily responsibilities						
Grade School	2.2	3.9	26.5	22.5	45.7	24.5
High School	(2.3)	(2.8)	(31.3)	(23.7)	(58.0)	(26.5)
College	1.2	4.3	35.5	28.3	63.6	28.9
No answer						
Grade School	8.0	7.1	9.4	8.2	8.2	7.3
High School	(1.0)	(1.2)	(3.1)	(.7)	(1.0)	(.7)
College	2.3	1.4	2.6	2.3	2.6	1.7

* N = 240 for Grade School Group, 392 for High School Group, and 163 for College Group.

TABLE 8

Per Cent of Responses by Illness Condition Regarding Information for Education Groups

Response and Education Group*	Critical	Worse	Not Up to Par	Better	Controlled	Chronic
Don't know						
Grade School	6.1	3.9	7.4	4.7	8.1	6.9
High School	(2.9)	(1.7)	(5.5)	(1.7)	(3.3)	(2.6)
College	1.4	2.9	10.1	4.6	6.4	2.6
Make sure that he tells you about any changes in his condition						
Grade School	55.9	39.6	19.4	18.6	18.4	15.1
High School	(60.4)	(50.4)	(19.6)	(25.4)	(17.3)	(24.2)
College	71.7	52.3	20.2	15.3	13.6	12.4
Encourage him to tell you about any change in his condition						
Grade School	21.4	36.5	27.0	21.4	20.6	24.3
High School	(30.8)	(40.5)	(29.7)	(23.6)	(22.3)	(25.9)
College	23.4	40.2	32.1	35.3	23.1	27.7
Discourage him from bothering you about every ache and pain						
Grade School	3.1	2.7	19.6	25.9	24.3	27.2
High School	(2.6)	(1.1)	(21.2)	(25.4)	(26.0)	(20.0)
College	.6	1.7	20.8	44.2	29.5	30.9
Steer him away from bothering you about every ache and pain						
Grade School	3.7	7.8	15.9	20.8	18.1	16.4
High School	(1.6)	(4.6)	(21.8)	(22.4)	(29.5)	(25.6)
College	1.2	1.4	15.0	25.1	24.9	24.9
No answer						
Grade School	9.8	9.4	10.6	8.6	10.4	10.0
High School	(1.6)	(1.7)	(2.0)	(1.4)	(1.7)	(1.6)
College	1.7	1.4	1.7	1.4	2.4	1.4

* N = 240 for Grade School Group, 392 for High School Group, and 163 for College Group.

TABLE 9

Per Cent of Responses by Illness Condition Regarding Medical Care for Low-, Middle- and High-Income Groups

Response and Income Group*	Critical	Worse	Not Up to Par	Better	Con-trolled	Chronic
Don't know						
Low	0.7	0.3	2.4	2.8	8.2	2.4
Middle	(.7)	(1.0)	(1.0)	(5.3)	(8.2)	(2.4)
High	—	—	—	11.3	16.9	.9
See to it that he sees a doctor						
Low	69.2	33.2	26.3	18.3	15.3	26.4
Middle	(75.0)	(41.8)	(23.6)	(12.1)	(11.2)	(28.4)
High	78.7	42.6	22.6	6.1	5.6	23.5
Encourage him to see a doctor						
Low	21.9	60.2	56.0	27.6	25.4	38.6
Middle	(20.7)	(55.3)	(65.4)	(37.2)	(28.3)	(44.2)
High	18.3	56.5	75.6	30.0	22.6	45.2
Discourage him from running to a doctor with small aches and pains						
Low	1.7	1.7	4.7	31.3	25.6	17.6
Middle	(.9)	(.3)	(4.9)	(30.0)	(34.5)	(15.7)
High	.4	—	—	39.1	35.7	20.0
See to it that he doesn't run to a doctor with small aches and pains						
Low	2.4	.9	6.1	16.0	20.5	11.3
Middle	(1.1)	(.7)	(3.9)	(13.5)	(18.7)	(8.3)
High	.9	.9	1.7	13.5	18.7	10.4
No answer						
Low	4.0	3.6	4.5	4.0	5.0	3.6
Middle	(1.6)	(.9)	(3.9)	(1.9)	(1.9)	(.9)
High	1.7	—	—	—	.4	—

* N = 272 for Low Group, 327 for Middle Group, and 108 for High Group.

TABLE 10

Per Cent of Responses by Illness Condition Regarding Physical Comfort for Low-, Middle- and High-Income Groups

Response and Income Group*	Critical	Worse	Not Up to Par	Better	Con-trolled	Chronic
Don't know						
Low	1.2	.3	7.8	3.7	3.3	1.4
Middle	(1.1)	(2.0)	(8.9)	(1.3)	(1.6)	(1.4)
High	.4	1.7	7.8	.4	2.6	2.2
Give them a great deal of extra care						
Low	65.6	68.9	19.6	9.7	13.0	17.6
Middle	(71.3)	(63.6)	(15.9)	(4.6)	(9.5)	(16.8)
High	74.3	64.3	15.2	5.6	7.8	6.9
See to it that they are comfortable						
Low	23.6	19.5	21.0	25.0	12.5	34.9
Middle	(23.4)	(28.0)	(22.7)	(20.0)	(6.7)	(35.5)
High	22.6	25.7	24.8	23.9	8.7	46.5
Encourage them to do things for themselves						
Low	2.1	4.3	21.2	46.8	31.5	22.4
Middle	(.6)	(2.9)	(19.7)	(62.3)	(25.9)	(26.9)
High	.9	4.3	16.1	59.1	26.5	24.8
Treat them like everybody else						
Low	1.4	2.1	23.3	12.2	33.6	17.0
Middle	(2.0)	(2.6)	(29.6)	(11.3)	(54.7)	(18.4)
High	.9	3.9	33.0	10.9	53.5	19.1
No answer						
Low	6.1	4.9	7.0	5.6	6.1	6.6
Middle	(1.6)	(.9)	(3.2)	(.4)	(1.6)	(1.0)
High	.9	—	3.0	—	.9	.4

* N = 272 for Low Group, 327 for Middle Group, and 108 for High Group.

Per Cent of Responses by Illness Condition Regarding Social Responsibility for Low-, Middle- and High-Income Groups

Response and Income Group*	Critical	Worse	Not Up to Par	Better	Controlled	Chronic
Don't know						
Low	2.4	3.1	8.2	1.2	5.6	5.4
Middle	(2.3)	(2.6)	(9.3)	(1.3)	(3.2)	(3.7)
High	1.3	2.2	8.3	1.7	3.9	2.6
Make major decisions for them						
Low	34.3	10.8	8.5	6.6	3.6	8.7
Middle	(40.9)	(11.3)	(5.7)	(2.6)	(2.7)	(4.9)
High	43.0	9.1	4.8	1.7	.9	4.9
Keep responsibilities and worries from them						
Low	46.9	67.1	26.1	16.9	7.1	21.9
Middle	(52.4)	(73.4)	(24.8)	(12.3)	(7.9)	(19.1)
High	52.2	73.5	22.6	12.6	9.6	20.0
Encourage them to do some sort of useful work						
Low	5.9	11.1	22.8	49.7	28.9	34.8
Middle	(1.6)	(7.0)	(25.3)	(55.0)	(24.1)	(42.1)
High	1.7	7.8	20.1	51.2	25.6	41.7
Urge them to carry their daily responsibilities						
Low	3.3	1.6	27.3	18.3	47.5	22.9
Middle	(1.7)	(4.3)	(32.2)	(28.2)	(61.3)	(29.7)
High	—	5.6	33.9	30.0	58.7	33.0
No answer						
Low	7.1	6.3	7.1	7.3	7.3	6.3
Middle	(1.0)	(.9)	(2.6)	(.6)	(.7)	(.4)
High	1.7	1.7	4.3	2.2	2.2	1.7

* N = 272 for Low Group, 327 for Middle Group, and 108 for High Group.

TABLE 12

Per Cent of Responses by Illness Condition Regarding Information For Low-, Middle- and High-Income Groups

Response and Income Group*	Critical	Worse	Not Up to Par	Better	Controlled	Chronic
Don't know						
Low	4.2	1.9	4.5	2.1	5.4	3.1
Middle	(3.6)	(2.9)	(8.6)	(2.1)	(4.3)	(4.0)
High	1.3	1.3	9.6	6.1	8.3	3.5
Make sure that he tells you about any change in his condition						
Low	49.4	41.7	20.0	27.5	17.2	20.7
Middle	(63.4)	(54.4)	(17.2)	(18.2)	(17.7)	(18.5)
High	79.1	47.4	20.4	11.3	9.1	13.5
Encourage him to tell you about any change in his condition						
Low	30.9	38.4	27.8	17.4	22.9	25.7
Middle	(28.6)	(36.8)	(31.8)	(33.8)	(23.4)	(27.3)
High	15.2	45.2	27.4	27.8	18.7	21.7
Discourage him from bothering you about every ache and pain						
Low	3.8	2.4	21.2	26.6	23.3	20.2
Middle	(1.1)	(1.3)	(23.4)	(23.4)	(27.3)	(26.6)
High	1.3	2.2	16.1	19.1	30.0	26.1
Steer him away from bothering you about every ache and pain						
Low	2.8	7.5	18.8	18.4	22.9	22.2
Middle	(2.4)	(2.9)	(16.9)	(21.8)	(25.4)	(22.1)
High	1.3	2.2	23.5	33.9	31.7	33.5
No answer						
Low	8.7	8.0	7.6	8.0	8.2	8.2
Middle	(.8)	(1.7)	(2.0)	(.6)	(1.7)	(1.4)
High	1.7	1.7	3.0	1.7	2.2	1.7

* N = 272 for Low Group, 337 for Middle Group, and 108 for High Group

TABLE 13

Per Cent of Responses by Income Group to Statements about What a Person Can Do When Sick at Home

Statement	Under $4,000 (N=272)	$4,000–$7,499 (N=327)	$7,500 and over (N=108)
1. When a person is sick, he is helpless	15.1	8.2	3.5
2. There is very little he can do for himself	22.0	13.5	8.7
3. He can still do some things for himself	43.5	55.6	65.2
4. He can still do most things for himself	13.9	20.9	19.6
Don't know; no answer	5.5	1.7	3.1

TABLE 14

Per Cent of Responses by Income Group to Statements about Doctors and Patients

Statement	Under $4,000 (N=272)	$4,000–$7,499 (N=327)	$7,500 and over (N=108)
1. Not much sense in strictly following doctor's orders; will get well anyway	0.7	0.3	1.7
2. Sick person can only do so much; it's up to doctor to get him well	22.7	17.7	13.0
3. All doctor can do is give instructions; it's up to the patient	68.8	77.6	81.7
4. Sick person knows better than doctor what's wrong	4.3	2.9	2.2
Don't know; no answer	3.5	1.5	1.3

TABLE 15

Per Cent of Responses by Income Group to Statements about What Happens When a Person is Sick at Home

Statement	Under $4,000 (N=272)	$4,000–$7,499 (N=327)	$7,500 and over (N=108)
1. His family will leave him out of things	7.2	4.0	4.8
2. His family will keep worries and problems from him	58.3	64.2	68.2
3. Family still counts on him to carry out duties and obligations	8.3	15.1	15.6
4. Family will make no important decisions without his OK	19.8	15.6	10.9
Don't know; no answer	6.4	1.0	5.2

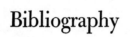

Bibliography

Bibliography

APPLE, DORRIAN. "How Laymen Define Illness," *Journal of Health and Human Behavior*, I (Fall, 1960), 219–25.

———— (ed.). *Sociological Studies of Health and Sickness.* New York: McGraw-Hill Book Co., 1960.

BARBER, BERNARD. "Structural–functional Analysis," *American Sociological Review*, XXI (April, 1956), 129–35.

BARNES, HARRY ELMER. *An Introduction to the History of Sociology.* Chicago: University of Chicago Press, 1948.

BATES, FREDERICK L. "A Conceptual Analysis of Group Structure," *Social Forces*, XXXVI (December, 1957), 103–11.

————. "Position, Role, and Status: A Reformulation of Concepts," *Social Forces*, XXXIV (May, 1956), 313–21.

BAUMANN, BARBARA. "Diversities in Conceptions of Health and Physical Fitness," *Journal of Health and Human Behavior*, II (Spring, 1961), 39–46.

BEN-DAVID, J. "The Professional Role of the Physician in Bureaucratized Medicine," *Human Relations*, XI (1958), 255–74.

BIDWELL, CHARLES E. "Some Effects of Administrative Behavior: A Study in Role Theory," *Administrative Science Quarterly*, II (1957), 163–81.

BLAU, PETER M. "Formal Organization: Dimensions of Analysis," *American Journal of Sociology*, LXIII (1957), 58–69.

BORING, E. G. "Psychology," *Encyclopaedia Britannica* (1952 ed.), XVIII, 675.

BROWN, ESTHER LUCILE. *Newer Dimensions of Patient Care.* New York: Russell Sage Foundation, 1961.

CAMERON, NORMAN. *The Psychology of Behavior Disorders—A Biosocial Interpretation.* Boston: Houghton Mifflin Co., 1947.

CHINOY, ELY. *Society.* New York: Random House, 1961.

COSER, ROSE L. "Authority and Decision-making in a Hospital: A Comparative Analysis," *American Sociological Review,* XXIII (February, 1958), 58–63.

DAVIS, KINGSLEY. *Human Society.* New York: Macmillan Co., 1949.

————. "The Myth of Functional Analysis as a Special Method in Sociology and Anthropology," *American Sociological Review,* XXIV (December, 1959), 757–72.

DURKHEIM, EMILE. *Suicide.* Glencoe, Ill.: Free Press, 1951.

EYSENCK, H. J. "Primary Social Attitudes—A Comparison of Attitude Patterns in England, Germany and Sweden," *Journal of Abnormal and Social Psychology,* XLVIII (1953), 563–68.

FREEMAN, HOWARD E. "Attitude toward Mental Illness," *American Sociological Review,* XXVI (February, 1961), 59–66.

FREEMAN, HOWARD E., and SIMMONS, OZZIE G. "Mental Patients in the Community: Family Settings and Performance Levels," *American Sociological Review,* XXIII (1958), 147–54.

FREIDSON, ELIOT. *Patients' Views of Medical Practice.* New York: Russell Sage Foundation, 1961.

GILLIAM, SYLVIA B., DEGROOT, IDA, and MARX, JOHN H. "Operationalization of the Theoretical Framework for the Study of Patterns of Medical Care," Working Paper, New York City Department of Health (mimeographed).

GILLIN, JOHN (ed.). *For a Science of Social Man.* New York: Macmillan Co., 1954.

GOODE, WILLIAM J. "Norm Commitment and Conformity to Role Status Obligations," *American Journal of Sociology,* LXVI (November, 1960), 246–58.

GROSS, N., MASON, W. S., and McEACHERN, A. W. *Explorations in Role Analysis.* New York: John Wiley & Sons, Inc., 1958.

JACO, E. GARTLY (ed.). *Patients, Physicians and Illness.* Glencoe, Ill.: Free Press, 1958.

KASSELBAUM, GENE G., and BAUMANN, BARBARA. "Dimensions of the Sick Role." Cornell University Medical College, March, 1960 (mimeographed).

LEVINSON, DANIEL J. "Role, Personality, and Social Structure in the Organizational Setting," *Journal of Abnormal and Social Psychology*, LVIII (March, 1959), 170–80.

LINDZEY, GARDNER (ed.). *Handbook of Social Psychology*. Cambridge: Addison-Wesley Publishing Co., 1954.

LINTON, RALPH. *The Study of Man*. New York: D. Appleton-Century Co., 1936.

LOOMIS, CHARLES P. *Social Systems*. Princeton: D. Van Nostrand Co., 1960.

MANGRIS, A. R. "Role Theory and Marriage Counseling," *Social Forces*, XXXV (March, 1957), 200–209.

MEAD, GEORGE HERBERT. *Mind, Self, and Society*. Chicago: University of Chicago Press, 1952.

MECHANIC, DAVID. "The Concept of Illness Behavior," *Journal of Chronic Diseases*, XV (February, 1962), 189–94.

MECHANIC, DAVID, and VOLKART, EDMUND A. "Stress, Illness, and the Sick Role," *American Sociological Review*, XXVI (February, 1961), 51–58.

MERTON, ROBERT K. "The Role-Set: Problems in Sociological Theory," *British Journal of Sociology*, VIII (1957), 106–20.

MERTON, ROBERT K., BROOM, LEONARD, and COTTRELL, LEONARD S., JR. (eds.). *Sociology Today*. New York: Basic Books, Inc., 1959.

MILLS, C. WRIGHT. *The Sociological Imagination*. New York: Oxford University Press, 1959.

NEIMAN, LIONEL J., and HUGHES, JAMES W. "The Problem of the Concept of Role—A Survey of the Literature," *Social Forces*, XXX (December, 1951), 141–49.

NETT, EMILY M. "Some Social and Psychological Correlates of Attitudes toward Medical Doctors. (Paper presented at the annual meeting of American Sociological Society, Washington, D.C., August, 1957, mimeographed.)

NEWCOMB, THEODORE M. *Social Psychology*. New York: Dryden Press, 1951.

PARSONS, TALCOTT. *The Social System*. Glencoe, Ill.: Free Press, 1951.

SARBIN, THEODORE R. "Role Theory," *Handbook of Social Psychology*, edited by Gardner Lindzey. Cambridge, Mass.: Addison-Wesley Publishing Co., 1954.

SAUNDERS, LYLE. *Cultural Difference and Medical Care.* New York: Russell Sage Foundation, 1954.

SWANSON, G. E., NEWCOMB, T. M., and HARTLEY, E. L. *Readings in Social Psychology.* New York: Henry Holt & Co., 1952.

TURNER, RALPH H. "Role-taking, Role Standpoint, and Reference-Group Behavior, *American Journal of Sociology,* LXI (January, 1956), 316–28.

ZOLA, IRVING K. "Socio-cultural Factors in the Seeking of Medical Aid." Massachusetts General Hospital (mimeographed).

Index

Aims of this investigation, 45
Analysis, methods of, 105-21
Anthropologists, treatment of role
  by, 22-24
Apple, Dorrian, 39, 41, 49, 50, 76,
  79, 151
Attitudes regarding illness and sick
  role, questions on, 45-46

Barber, Bernard, 151
Barnes, Harry Elmer, 27, 151
Bates, Frederick L., 30-33, 151
Baumann, Barbara, 41, 151, 152
Bed, "sick" responses and confine-
  ment to, 57
Behavioral expectations
  in illness, 71-96
  regarding ill person, 42-44, 71-92
    effect of socioeconomic status
      on, 83-85
  regarding role relationships of
    sick person, 92-96
  and socioeconomic status, 99
Behavioral presumptions of sick role,
  36-37
Ben-David, J., 151
Bidwell, Charles E., 151
Blau, Peter M., 151
Boring, E. G., 151
Broom, Leonard, 39, 153
Brown, Esther Lucile, 151

Cameron, Norman, 26, 152
Chinoy, Ely, 31, 152
Chronic illness (*see also* Functional
  incapacity)
  common element in Cluster 2, 53
Cluster analysis
  Clusters *1-4*, 52-53
  Clusters *5-6*, 76-91
  of dyadic role relationships, 94
  use of, in this study, 112-13
Comte, I. Auguste, 27

Coser, Rose, 39, 152
Cottrell, Leonard S., Jr., 39, 153

Davis, Allison, 80
Davis, Kingsley, 29, 31, 152
DeGroot, Ida, 41, 152
Demographic data obtained, 46
Dependency of ill person, 43-44, 72-
  75, 77-85
  and low- and high-status groups,
    100
  and role relationships, 92-96
Doctor
  care by
    as criterion of status sick, 50
    and dependency of ill person,
      72-75, 78, 84-89, 108
    and "sick" responses, 56
      of low- and high-status
        groups, 69-70
      relation between socioeco-
        nomic status and, 42
      of three income groups, 63
  obligation of, to prescribe social
    response to ill person, 100-1
Durkheim, Emile, 27, 152
Dyadic role relationships, 43-44, 93-
  96, 109

Education
  and behavioral expectations re-
    garding ill person, 85-90
  and responses concerning dyadic
    role relationships, 95-96
  and "sick" responses, 63-70
Eysenck, H. J., 47, 152

Freeman, Howard E., 152
Freidson, Eliot, 35, 38, 40, 152
Functional incapacity
  and behavioral expectations re-
    garding ill person, 75-76, 91-
    92

common element in Cluster *1*, 53
as criterion of status sick, 42-43,
    50, 55-57, 60-63
and "sick" responses
    of groups classified by income
        and education, 64-70
    of persons in three income
        groups, 60-63
    and socioeconomic status as fac-
        tors in "sick" responses, 42-
        43, 99

Gilliam, Sylvia B., 41, 152
Gillin, John, 23, 29, 152
Goode, William J., 32, 152
Gross, N., 23, 24, 32, 33, 39, 152

Hartley, E. L., 80, 154
Hughes, James W., 24, 153
Hypotheses tested, 42-44
    and relevant questionnaire items,
        106-11
    and statistical techniques, 106-10
    validity of, 97-98
    Nos. *1-3*, 70
    Nos. *4-6*, 91
    Nos. *7-8*, 96

Ill person
    behavioral expectations regarding,
        71-92
    dependency of, 43-44, 72-75, 78,
        84-89, 92-96, 100
    responses expected from him and
        for him, 72-73
    role relationships and behavioral
        expectations regarding, 92-96
Illness
    attitudes regarding, 45-46
    behavioral expectations in, 42-44
    conditions of
        correlations of responses to, 77-
            78
        descriptions of, 50-51
        variation in responses to, 79-
            81
    dependence and independence in,
        43-44

Impaired role
    behavioral expectations regarding,
        99-101
    defined by behavioral expecta-
        tions, 77
    responses toward and from per-
        son occupying, 77-79
Incapacity, *see* Functional incapac-
    ity
Income groups (*see also* Socioeco-
    nomic status)
    responses of, to illness conditions,
        81-90
    "sick" responses of, 58-70
Individual, the, and role, 24-27
Information supplied by ill person
    and dependency, 72-75, 78, 84-
        89, 109
Interviewing
    excerpts from manual on, 113-15
    techniques in, 46-47

Jaco, E. Gartley, 39, 152
James, William, 25

Kasselbaum, Gene G., 41, 152
Koos, Earl Lomon, 41, 79

Lazarsfeld, Paul F., 28
Legitimization of illness by physi-
    cian, *see* Doctor, care by
Levinson, Daniel J., 21, 32, 153
Lindzey, Gardner, 25, 153
Linton, Ralph, 23, 24, 153
Loomis, Charles P., 28, 29, 41, 153

McClelland, David C., 26
McEachern, A. W., 23, 24, 32, 33,
    39, 152
Mangris, A. R., 153
Marx, John H., 41, 152
Mason, W. S., 23, 24, 32, 33, 39,
    152
Mead, George Herbert, 25-27, 153
Mechanic, David, 39, 49, 50, 76, 153
Medical care, *see* Doctor, care by
Merton, Robert K., 39, 153
Mills, C. Wright, 28, 29, 153
Murdock, George P., 23
Murphy, Gardner, 25

Neiman, Lionel J., 24, 153
Nett, Emily M., 41, 153
Newcomb, Theodore M., 26, 80, 153, 154

Parsons, Talcott, 17, 22, 25, 27, 29, 35, 36-39, 40-42, 42-44, 45, 71-72, 76, 91, 92, 93, 94, 97, 99, 107, 109, 153
Personality and role, 26-27
Persons interviewed, 47
Physical comfort and dependency of ill person, 72-75, 78, 84-89, 108-9
Physical incapacity, *see* Functional incapacity
Physician, *see* Doctor
Prognosis
   and behavioral expectations regarding ill person, 42-44, 72-76
   as criterion of status sick, 50
   as determinant of behavioral expectations in sick role, 91-92
   and responses by income groups to illness conditions, 81-85
   and "sick" responses, 42-43, 55-57
      of groups classified by income, 59-63
      of groups classified by income and education, 64-70
   and socioeconomic status as factors in "sick" responses, 99
Psychologist, treatment of role by, 24-27

Questionnaire used in interviewing, 45-46
   items of, relevant to hypotheses, 106-11
   order and methods of presentation of items on, 116-21

Reciprocal relationship in sociological analysis, 28-32
Recovering from illness, common element in Cluster 3, 53
Research
   design of this investigation, 45-47

   procedures in this investigation, 105-21
Role
   concept of, 21, 38-41
   and individual behavior, 24-27
   and personality, 26-27
   the sick (*see also* Sick role, the), 35-43
   and sociology, 27-33
   and status, 30-32
   theory of, 21-33
   treatment of, by anthropologists, 22-24
   treatment of, by psychologists, 24-27
   unimodal conceptions of, 38-41
Role expectations in illness states, cause of differences in, 99
Role relationships
   dyadic, 43-44
   in sickness, 36
   of sick person, 92-96
Role response, importance of, to ill person's progress, 100-1

Sampling procedure used in this investigation, 47, 105-6
Sarbin, Theodore R., 25, 26, 27, 153
Sargent, Steven Stansfeld, 26
Saunders, Lyle, 41, 80, 154
Shils, Edward A., 25
"Sick" and "not sick" responses to given descriptions of illness, 54-57
Sick person, *see* Ill person
Sick person–doctor relationship, 43 92-96, 99
Sick person–family relationship, 43, 93-96, 99
Sick person–self relationship, 43, 92-96
Sick role, the, 35-43
   behavioral expectations regarding, 99-101
   behavioral presumptions of, 36-37
   concept of
      need for evaluation of, 97
      useful in social analysis, 35
   defined by behavioral expectations, 77

reactions in rejection of, 38
responses to and from person occupying, 77-79
sociological orientation in study of, 33
as a sociological variable, 39-40
Sick status, *see* Status sick
Simmons, Ozzie G., 152
Social environment and treatment of ill person, 100-1
Social responsibility and dependency of ill person, 72-75, 78, 84-89, 109
Socioeconomic status (*see also* Income groups)
   and doctor's care in identification of status sick, 42
   and education, effect of, on responses to illness conditions, 85-90
   and identification of status sick, 57-70
   and physical incapacities in identification of status sick, 42-44
   and responses concerning dyadic role relationships, 94-96
   and responses to illness conditions, 79-90
   variations in responses of groups occupying different, 98-99
Sociological Abstracts, 39
Sociologist, treatment of role by, 27-33
Sorokin, Pitirim A., 29
Spencer, Herbert, 27

Statistical procedures, 106-13
Status and role, 22-24, 30-32
Status groups, low and high
   defined, 67
   and dependency of ill person, 100
   responses of, to illness conditions, 87-91
   "sick" responses of, 67-70
Status sick
   correlations of factors used for validating, 52-53
   criteria for validating, 49-70
   factors important in validating, 50
   hypotheses concerning, 42-44
Sullivan, Harry Stack, 26
Swanson, G. E., 80, 154
Symptomatology
   as criterion of status sick, 50, 63, 70
   and "sick" responses, 56

Tables, source
   for Chapter IV, 125-32
   for Chapter V, 135-48
Turner, Ralph H., 32, 154

Volkart, Edmund A., 39, 153

Weber, Max, 27
Work, ability to
   common element in Cluster 4, 53
   and "sick" responses, 57

Zola, Irving K., 40, 154